Creativity and the Dissociative Patient

of related interest

Art Therapy, Race and Culture
Edited by Jean Campbell, Marian Liebmann, Frederica Brooks, Jenny Jones and Cathy Ward
ISBN 1 85302 578 X pb
ISBN 1 85302 579 8 hb

Tapestry of Cultural Issues in Art Therapy
Edited by Anna Hiscox and Abby Calisch
ISBN 1 85302 576 3 pb

Reflections on Therapeutic Storymaking
The Use of Stories in Groups
Alida Gersie
ISBN 1 85302 272 1 pb

Arts Approaches to Conflict
Edited by Marian Liebmann
ISBN 1 85302 293 4

Creativity and the Dissociative Patient
Puppets, Narrative and Art in the Treatment of Survivors of Childhood Trauma

Lani Alaine Gerity

Preface by Edith Kramer

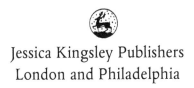

Jessica Kingsley Publishers
London and Philadelphia

First published in the United Kingdom in 1999 by
Jessica Kingsley Publishers
116 Pentonville Road
London N1 9JB, UK
and
400 Market Street, Suite 400
Philadelphia, PA19106, USA.

www.jkp.com

Copyright © Lani Alaine Gerity 1999
Printed digitally since 2002

Library of Congress Cataloging in Publication Data
Gerity, Lani Alaine, 1953–
Creativity and the dissociative patient : puppets, narrative, and
art in the treatment of survivors of childhood trauma / Lani Alaine Gerity.
p. cm. Includes bibliographical references and index.
ISBN 1-85302-722-7 (pb : alk. paper)
1. Dissociative disorders – Treatment. 2. Puppets – Therapeutic
use. I. Title. RC553.D5G47 1999
616.85'23065156--dc21 98-42739
CIP

British Library Cataloguing in Publication Data
Gerity, Lani Alaine,
Creativity and the dissociative patient : puppets, narrative, and art in the treatment of
survivors of childhood trauma
1. Art therapy 2. Puppet making – Therapeutic use
I. Title
616.8'91656

ISBN-13: 978 1 85302 722 2
ISBN-10: 1 85302 722 7

Contents

ACKNOWLEDGEMENTS 6

PREFACE BY EDITH KRAMER 9

1. Introduction 13
Population and Agents of Change

2. The Case of Jenny 23

3. Object Relations Theories and Application 63

4. Metaphor and Story 87
'Anything Can Happen in Puppetland'

5. Transference and Splitting 97
The Abyss – Self and Community

6. Healing the Split 105
Margaret, Winter Solstice and the Monster

7. Reparation and the Wise Old Woman 115
The Conclusion

Postscript 123
Tying Up Loose Ends

REFERENCES 135

SUBJECT INDEX 145

AUTHOR INDEX 149

Acknowledgements

I would like to acknowledge my debt and gratitude to all my teachers, family, and friends. Not being able to thank everyone individually for everything they have done, I will have to pick a few from the many to acknowledge.

Jenny and all of the passionate artists that I have had the honor of working with were very patient and inspiring teachers. Of my many instructors at New York University, I am particularly grateful to those who advised and guided the dissertation that preceded this book: Professor Laurie Wilson, Professor Robert Landy, and most especially Professor Edith Kramer for reading through this material so carefully, and gently pointing out how Kleinian language pathologizes normal developmental stages and inspite of that wrote such a wonderful preface.

I would also like to thank Laura Silverstein for her support and advice. For my friends who listened to all of the puppet stories that came out of this work, thank you. Toby, without your curiosity about theory during those long evening discussions, I would never have thought of putting it on paper.

I am indebted to my entire family for their encouragement and interest, but especially to Edna for urging me on during the more difficult times and to Edward for listening to endless permutations of thought and always asking the right questions and just because.

In memory of William Gerity Jr.

Preface

As the title tells us, this complex, very rich and charming book describes an art therapist's work with survivors of childhood trauma that included sexual abuse, desertion and assault, resulting in chronic mental illness. The survivors were clients of a large day treatment center in New York City.

Dr Ernst Federn, psychoanalytically trained psychotherapist once explained to me that there are three major kinds of emotional disturbances. First, there are individuals whose suffering is caused by repressed early childhood fantasies that continue to influence and disturb their adult lives. Second, there are those who suffer from the inability to distinguish between their inner world and the real world in which they must function. Finally, there are those who have been helpless victims of extreme physical and emotional cruelties, so that unendurable memories of these experiences intrude into their waking days, crippling their lives.

Jenny, the chief protagonist of Gerity's story, as well as most of the supporting patient-actors in the drama of Jenny's treatment belong to the third category. For these victims of childhood trauma, any verbal questioning, any attempt at gaining direct insight into their inner lives, is easily interpreted as yet another assault that must be warded off. Gerity had to devise treatment approaches that would not inflict injury in the name of therapy. As every therapist must, Gerity had to be aware of the double face of psychiatric symptoms. No matter how burdensome they may appear, they constitute the individuals defense against the full impact of psychic injury, preventing or forestalling more extensive mental breakdown. The therapist must approach symptoms cautiously and respectfully.

Jenny had grown up a battered child in hunger and poverty. There were indications that she had received a certain measure of loving care as an infant. However at three years of age she was despairing enough to attempt suicide by ingesting a bottle of aspirin. Throughout her childhood Mother had threatened to abandon her. Father had attempted to kill her when she was six years old. At that age she was also raped by a neighbor and molested by an uncle. Mother had failed to protect her against any of those assaults.

As an adult Jenny had dealt with her rage and pain as well as with her persistent longing for love from her cold and demanding mother by dissociating. She became three distinct personalities, a good humored personality who loved to sing, a destructive severely critical personality and Jenny, a child-like dependent individual. It requires high intelligence, creative imagination and a strong will to create and maintain several distinct personalities. The therapist must respect the patient's achievement and must neither denigrate these several personalities nor express doubt that they indeed exist.

It's one of the charms of this book that the reader is not presented with a cut and dry case history followed by an account of the subsequent treatment. Rather, Lani Gerity allows us to follow her, as she is puzzled by the radical and mysterious changes in Jenny's moods and behavior. At this junction, we learn of Jenny's childhood and of her several identities.

Within the realm of art therapy at the center, two activities proved particularly helpful to Jenny. Work with clay, a forgiving material that can endure endless doing and undoing, absorb destructive cutting and poking and still permit the making of well integrated handsome sculptural work. Jenny develops great skill in making pots, slab-constructions and sculptures. The activity calms and reassures her. In the pottery room Jenny is able to work independently.

Puppetry involves a number of patients, Gerity, drama therapist and student interns, and puppets, which the participants create and animate. This group has playful aspects, but it is distinct from children's imaginative play where everything is fluid and subject to change. The dramas enacted by the patients' puppets are structured, they endure and evolve over weeks and months much as the puppets themselves endure and evolve. They are taken seriously and deal with deeply felt emotions and perplexities. Art therapists are familiar with the power of visual image to symbolically give form to unbearable and unspeakable material. We find that these puppets have the power to talk about many things that would not otherwise be permitted verbal expression. Criticism as well as encouragement that would fall on deaf ears or arouse anger if it came from a therapist or a fellow patient can be heard and integrated when a puppet speaks.

Evidently Lani Gerity's creative imagination, her profound involvement, indeed her belief in Puppetland makes it come alive, makes it profoundly moving and fascinating for the patients and the reader.

Yet Gerity never allows herself to get lost in Puppetland to the extent of forgetting her function as the puppeteer's therapist. Accounts of winter solstice ceremonies for puppets and of fairy tale readings alternate with theoretical passages where Gerity discusses child development, loss, and reparation as seen by clinicians and theoretical thinkers as Melanie Klein, Margaret Mahler, Winnicott, Shengold and others. Eventually Jenny becomes an integrated individual. The split is healed.

She begins to separate from the center. Jenny's emotional health is, however, paid for by physical impairment. Here again we must admire Gerity's courage to admit that success and failure interlock. As we all know, but sometimes try to forget, psychotherapy heals the healthy and supports the sick. It alleviates their suffering but is powerless to entirely eliminate deeply anchored pathology.

We leave Jenny conducting her life from her wheelchair. She applies what she has learned at the center. She is the art lady of her housing project and she has also set up a home nursing service where she acts as a go-between, providing understanding and encouraging cooperation between patients and nurses.

I find that my introduction has turned into a synopsis of Gerity's book. I hope that it has merely stimulated the desire to learn more about Jenny, puppetry and dissociation in this unusual and absorbing book.

Professor Edith Kramer,
Art Therapy Program, New York University; Visiting Professor, George Washington University
Author of Art As Therapy with Children *and* Childhood and Art Therapy
March 1999

CHAPTER I

Introduction

Population and Agents of Change

This book contains the lessons learned while working for more than a decade as an art therapist in a large mental health day treatment center in Manhattan. During this time I had the opportunity to work with many people who fell within a wide range of diagnostic categories, in both individual and group setting, in art therapy groups as well as verbal groups. It was possible to see what appeared to be correlations between diagnosis and preferences toward specific modalities of treatment.

The clients most drawn to art therapy seemed to have certain things in common. These included diagnoses of borderline personality disorder, dissociative identity disorder (formerly multiple personality disorder), or post traumatic stress disorder. In addition, their early histories tended to include various kinds of trauma or abuse. It seemed that these individuals were more open to art therapy than the more traditional verbal therapy. Because I had run both kinds of groups and could see it wasn't the therapist's personality that clients were reacting to, I couldn't help but wonder what it was about the nature of art therapy that drew them with such intensity. I thought if I could work with an individual closely and examine the art work that emerged, I might be better able to understand how and why art therapy works with this extremely difficult population. I might learn how and why they seemed to immerse themselves in the language and metaphor of art making with more facility than patients with other diagnoses. It seemed essential to know what in the art-making process was therapeutic for this population. A therapist determining this could fine-tune her treatment skills to meet the specific needs of the 'adult survivor'.

To that end this book includes a single case study of a dissociative patient, Jenny, who had a history of very severe early childhood trauma. Certain aspects of art therapy were of particular therapeutic value for her. For example, she found puppet making and puppet play to be especially beneficial. It seemed that the psychological concept of reparation was occurring as she pieced together various components to create a whole puppet, as if the external assemblage mirrored the process of psychological integration. Crucial to this process of integration was Jenny's role as puppeteer consciously orchestrating the cooperation and integration of her puppets/self. Another aspect of Jenny's treatment was the use of body image representations as a therapeutic intervention. While a healthy sense of self contains a cohesive body self, Jenny's development was compromised by abuse and trauma, resulting in a less than healthy, cohesive body self. Within art therapy Jenny was able to work on the development of a healthy sense of self by working with representations of body image.

In addition to Jenny's history and treatment, I would like to present some of the material, metaphors and stories, that emerged from other 'survivors' in a puppet-making group. By telling their stories, I hope to show how these individuals used what was in the art room to repair (or even generate in some cases) a cohesive, healthy, stronger sense of self and how this in turn led to a spirit of generosity and generativity within the community.

> ... the day I put my hands into the clay and started creating a head of a person who is very dear to me, something magical happened within me. I felt a deep connection to a deep part of myself. I could put all of myself into this clay – my love, my anger, my fears and create a thing of beauty. My soul could be validated in an object I could touch, feel, look at and feel a deep sense of self-worth and even self-love. And this, after all is the overall goal of my rehabilitation – to learn to cherish and love myself – from this everything else flows... when I created my clay head, I said, wow, I can do this. I didn't think I could. Maybe there are other things I can do.

> *48-year-old woman, survivor of childhood sexual abuse*

Changes come so slowly that they are very difficult to see. Progress used to seem unobtainable; because seeing beyond 'right now' requires a different vision, one that I never seemed to have before art. Five years ago, I was trapped in my mental illness – going from one doctor to another, so disabled by my own mind that I could no longer function in the outside world. I was desperate to break free, to find some way to let someone know how I felt, what was going on in my head. But I had no words. Then an art therapist gave me some clay, some pastels, paper – access to a world I had never known existed. And slowly, with her patience, and my determination to overcome my constant desire to just give up, I began to gain perspective, to see progress, to understand my mental illness and how I could use art to let others in to help me. At 30 years old, a time when I feel a lot of my peers are halfway through their lives, I have just begun my journey. The task of my healing is nothing less than arduous, undertaken in addition to my daily life. Through art, I am fighting my way back to reality and hope. Art is my window to your world, and yours to mine.

30-year-old woman, ritual cult survivor

Pottery lifts the spirit beyond any darkened shadow that covers a man's soul. I feel my spirit lift out of my illness re-firing my creative mind …

38-year-old man, survivor of childhood sexual abuse

These words were written by three individuals who were trying to express what they found of value in art therapy they received at the centre. As one of the art therapists working with these individuals, I was moved by their passion, but also curious. I wondered what it was about the nature of art therapy that these particular clients are so drawn to it.

The three clients above talked about the various ways that art therapy helped them. Working fairly closely with them, I had the opportunity to observe two things about these clients, who were fairly typical for this traumatized borderline–DID continuum. The first thing I observed was that they were very passionate and seemed better suited for the art room than for verbal groups where their passions seemed continually to get them into trouble. The second thing I noticed was that they seemed to use art materials in a reparative manner, but I will address this further along.

The population named 'chronically and persistently mentally ill' by the State of New York was the population our center treated. The persistence of their symptoms made them a difficult population. The survivors of early childhood trauma were, in our agency, a subgroup of this more general population, and because of their traumatic histories often had uniquely difficult interactions with staff. Their histories were often so horrific that the therapist could easily lose a sense of objectivity. In an effort to balance the perceived horror, staff might be tempted to treat the patients as very special. The well-meaning therapist may make every effort to counter the negative attention the patient received in childhood with positive attention. Sometimes the feeling was that all a particular patient needed was some love or affection, and that the therapist understood this where no one else ever did – indeed, often feeling, as one intern described, a 'special thread of understanding' between the patient and therapist. It was just this kind of singling out, or 'specialness', within the family structure that contributed to the problem of abuse or trauma. Such individuals are always alert to the behaviours of those they perceive as being 'in power'. They are alert and perhaps expectant. Unwittingly, the therapist may begin to treat the patients in exactly the manner that they expect. Often, very well-meaning therapists find themselves in positions of being a hated object and with such volatile, passionate individuals this can be extremely difficult.

In my observations, as you will soon see, creative arts therapists are fortunate to have objects and imagery to work with which often seem to absorb and drain off these excess passions. Objects and imagery become the focus for both patient and therapist. There is an investment of positive feelings in the 'transitional object' or the artwork and the transitional space, the actual place where the artwork is created. Because attention is not directly focused on the patient but rather on the productions, the patients often spoke of feeling safer in the art room or the pottery room than anywhere else in the building. Unwary art therapists and other staff might begin to think or believe that these positive feelings are caused by the art therapist's personality or her great efforts to understand the patient, leading to storms of countertransference. I suspected, however, that the facility these patients have in the creative arts and the feelings of safety that they express about the art room have less to do with the personality of the art therapist and have more to do with a fit between the needs of these individuals and the agents of change within the creative process.

But why look at the reparative qualities in art therapy, as seen specifically in the realm of body image? This was the second thing that I noticed about these patients, that they would often quite literally create various human body parts and make a whole of them, repairing the self-image or perhaps repairing the image of a loved one as quoted above. I think this can be best understood in terms of their histories of abuse, neglect and trauma to their bodily selves, how they carried physical memories which were reflected in their sense of self as a body. They expressed a feeling of being damaged, a feeling of being not an integrated whole body but a sum of odd, unrelated parts. One patient said she generally felt her left hand didn't know what her right hand was doing.

Interestingly, that feeling was recreated in the staff who worked with these patients, as if we were enacting their inner dramas. We could easily replicate the lack of integration among ourselves, in much the same way the patients would describe their inner worlds. Sometimes a therapist would simply find a patient intolerable and ask to have him or her removed from their group (usually a verbal group). Herman (1992) commented on this phenomenon, noting that adult survivors of childhood trauma 'evoke unusually intense reactions in caregivers' (p.123).

I became very interested in how this creative process unfolds, how the healing and reparative qualities of art therapy worked for this population. I wanted to understand the effects of childhood trauma as well as what helps these individuals and why. In understanding of how positive change occurs we also learn more about using our craft. These patients seemed to tolerate art groups, get along better with their peers in them, and even thrived in them, while continuing to be disruptive in verbal groups. It seemed that art therapy provided something that might not have been provided in any verbal modality. Is it that it engages the patient in reparative work on a preverbal level? Much of the trauma that occurred for these patients occurred before they had developed language, and it may be that having access to preverbal imagery is a particular strength of art therapy. Art therapy provided a place where the patient was able to return to the memory of early bodily traumas, now held within imagery, and provided the tools to express and *change* the meaning, intensity and intractability of the imagery. A patient was now able to begin to repair the damage done to his or her body image on a preverbal level, in a way that talking could never facilitate.

This book is about Jenny and a few other patients with similar passions and history of trauma. It is about their work to overcome the influence of the past in their present lives. Like many with a history of early childhood trauma, Jenny had a sense of self so fragmented that she gave names or labels to these various fragments, dissociated feelings and aspects of her personality (Carey, Joy and Jenny). Her artwork showed this same dissociation. Body image representations in the beginning of treatment were incomplete or in pieces, sometimes heads floating in space. Looking at body image representations to understand better the patient's sense of self is not a new idea.

Kramer (1993) stated that 'children's art is above all self representation' (p.79). She described evaluating a child's body image through his sculptures; a child who was reluctant to sculpt people, but 'the few attempts he could be induced to make proved that his body-image was intact and free from gross distortions' (p.79).

Krueger (1989) stated that the body image representation or projective drawing will be an arbitrary slice from the ongoing process of maturation, since one's body image evolves during one's life. He felt that in the course of successful therapy one can see clearly the process of maturation and distinctness of body image, paralleling developmental maturation. Concurring with these observations, I believe body image representation can be used as the measure of change, based on the hypothesis that it was an expression of the patient's sense of physical self. The body image representations of the people I worked with contained within them expressions of fragmentation, or pain, and then a sense of being soothed, or repaired, all of which will be shown later.

We will be examining a course of treatment, looking at the artwork produced and following the progress. Examining a course of treatment cannot be entirely objective since the author's personal bias is bound to influence the examination. Although research may be conducted rigorously and with care, therapists have to be particularly alert to bias introduced through the phenomena of transference and countertransference. Our day treatment center had its share of transference and countertransference issues, an ongoing factor in treatment, and of which many examples will follow. There were the patients' projections onto the art therapist as the good person providing art materials and the potential for reduction of stress, much as a good-enough mother would feed the child and reduce its stress. The verbal counselors often received negative projections because they were increasing the patients' anxiety and stress by verbal questioning, which was often experienced as prying or invasive, much as an abusive parent might invade a child's physical being and increases the child's stress. It was easier to experience empathy for the patients if one was the receptor of positive transferential feelings. At our agency, the patients' negative feelings towards those who were less than sympathetic towards them could be observed, as could the tension and controversy that occurred among staff when such transference and countertransference came to the fore.

Another aspect of subjectivity in this kind of book is the reality that as a therapist I had an investment in a successful outcome and thus was rarely simply a disinterested observer/writer. However, I found that a great deal can be learned from the therapist's reflection on the therapeutic process, the basis of a hermeneutic approach to learning.

The center

When Jenny arrived at the mental health day treatment center in the mid-1980s, it served 500 of New York City's chronically and persistently mentally ill population. This was the definition given by the State of New York in its Medicaid funding requirements. It lumped people together who, because of mental illness and their symptoms, couldn't maintain work and their place in society without support. These 500 patients came in for group therapy, individual therapy and to see a psychiatrist. At this time, the center was still psychodynamically based with a very creative team of drama, dance and art therapists who were responsible for most of the group work done there. During brainstorming sessions we would develop ideas for new groups, share some new creative idea that came from a conference, or suggest a new way of collaborating within a group. Of course, this was before our center began, for its survival, to look at fiscal concerns over and above other concerns. We still had a feeling of limitless possibilities at that time.

The center was housed in a former church with a small attached school building. The art room was converted from the pastor's study, complete with oak bookshelves, an oak window seat and leaded glass window panes. The free wall space was covered with particle boards which allowed patients to display as much of their artwork as possible without damaging the walls. All of the art supplies were accessible on the bookshelves, and we encouraged patients to take responsibility for the materials as well as for their artwork. We had one very large table that seated 15 people and one separate table for those who had difficulty being in a group.

A puppet-making group was held in the art room. The idea for this had come when I had observed a painfully shy young man complete a drawing of a beautiful woman and then take it to the full-length mirror, where he began playfully talking for it. Observing this, I asked questions of the picture and he easily answered through the picture, all signs of reticence having mysteriously disappeared. It was a light-hearted but, for me, exciting moment. It became clear that this reserved patient could more easily speak through a picture. The thought occurred to me that he and others might benefit from a puppet-making group where they could talk and play out various stories while working on body image representations.

During this time, there was also a separate room for pottery, complete with kiln, tools, clay and long tables at which several patients could work together. The pottery groups were run like open studio groups, less structured than art therapy, so patients could walk around the tables and talk to one another about work in progress. All in all, the program that was in place when Jenny arrived at our center had many creative options and possibilities for reparative work.

Defining reparation and body image

The term 'reparation' was used by Melanie Klein (1921) to indicate a psychological process, something more than the making of amends. She believed a young child will have many aggressive and sadistic feelings that she will project onto her environment. The child will then sense a need to create reparative gestures towards the damaged world in an effort to not be persecuted by it. As the reparative gestures reduce anxiety, feelings of guilt and constructive tendencies are able to come forward. With the patients like Jenny, though, it was much more than the world that had been damaged, it was their very selves that had been damaged and betrayed. These patients had internalized the traumata or abuse and continued to damage themselves. Clegg (1984, 1995) broadened the definition of reparation to include the self. He believed that gestures could be made towards the damaged world and towards the damaged self through various creative arts therapies turning this figurative gesture into something concrete. In our art room and pottery studio this repair of the damaged self could be seen in the integration of body image representations, thus for our purposes the term reparation will refer to the psychological process as well as its representation in the literal repairing of what has been damaged.

What do we mean by body image? For this discussion the term refers to the inner sensations and peripheral awareness that form the bodily experience of the individual. This would include the feelings and concepts that individuals have about their bodily experience which change and develop throughout their lives. Freud (1923) defined body image as a deposit of internalized images encompassing the self-representations and internalized representations of the loved object. Niederland (1967) described the concept of body image as being of central significance for the understanding of human personality growth. He saw body image as the felt experience of the body, the sum of personal, pervasive experiences which are derived from the interaction of postural, kinesthetic, physical functions with the sensorial, perceptive, emotional, cognitive functions. He proposed that it is this interaction which provides the coherent and cohesive backdrop for integrated ego functioning and for the development of gratifying object relations in later life.

From this we can easily see the importance of early bodily experience in the formation of human identity. If a patient had very negative early bodily experiences, she or he could easily develop a disintegrated sense of self, poor ego functioning, and would have impaired object relations in later life. But given the ability for feelings and concepts to change, reparative work was a very real possibility in our center with its strong creative arts program.

A note on the theoretical framework of this book

My clinical work has been most influenced or affected by the theories of Freud, Winnicott, Klein, as well as the current theorists, Ogden, Giovacchini, Grotstein and Bower, who discuss developmental disorders in terms of object relations, internalization and projective identification. Object relations theories speak to the issue of how we as humans develop a sense of who we are in the world. There is an acknowledgement of the fact that we internalize images of those who are important to our development, that we carry these images around with us and project them onto others and onto new situations. Object relations theorists focus on development of self through the internalization of images. They propose that we contain at our core images of what is and what was around us. It is through this collection of images and internalizations that we learn who we are. As a student of Edith Kramer and Laurie Wilson I was given a firm foundation in the healing potential of the creative act itself and I found that object relations theories shed some light on *why* the creative act is healing.

Art therapists working with individuals who have suffered early trauma can easily see these projections and internalizations because we have the luxury of being in a space which encourages the free expression and play of images and imagination. I found object relations theories satisfying in that they provide a way of examining and thinking about human development and imagery, a context and language with which to understand how humans create imagery and symbols. Moreover, they speak to questions of agents of change, thus I have relied heavily upon them as an explanatory model throughout the present analysis.

In addition to Jenny's history and treatment, I would like to present some of the material, metaphors and stories that emerged from other 'survivors' in the puppet-making group. By examining these stories in addition to Jenny's, I hope to follow the path these individuals took to repair (or even generate in some cases) a cohesive, healthy, stronger sense of self and how this in turn led to a spirit of generosity and generativity within the community, which presented a further layer of healing for these 'adult survivors'.

CHAPTER 2

The Case of Jenny

I began working with Jenny in September of 1985. Because of early childhood experiences, Jenny's sense of self was fragmented and inconsistent, but I didn't know her history or her changing sense of self when she first came to art therapy. My initial impression of this 40-year-old, 300-pound, African-American woman was of a simple, shy, childlike individual, a little frightened and somewhat clinging. In the art room, she always sat as close as possible to the door. When I would sit at the art table, I would also sit near the door to have a certain amount of influence over the comings and goings. I wasn't sure if Jenny wanted a quick escape route or access to the art therapist. Initially, her drawings were plain, little drawings of her environment, flowers and buildings done in a very childlike manner, over which she seemed compelled to always place barbed wire (Figure 2.1). This image of barbed wire repeated itself over and over, and was the first indication that perhaps Jenny's story was not as simple as it first appeared.

It was in the pottery studio that I observed Jenny's manner change. She exhibited excitement and enthusiasm. She didn't giggle shyly, but seemed more mature, more confident. She seemed to have more mastery over the materials when working with clay and, perhaps because of the mastery, more pleasure. She moved about the room easily, not needing to be at close proximity to an escape route or the art therapist. Typically, she would create breast-shaped containers that after much working and smoothing would become mugs. At first I dismissed this change of behavior as being related to Melanie Klein's theories about the breast; that somehow the pottery studio represented a source of 'comforts, physical and mental, an inexhaustible reservoir of food and warmth' (Segal 1964, p.40). In explaining Klein's theories, Segal states that there is a blissful experience of satisfaction that this wonderful object, the breast, can give and that the infant desires to possess

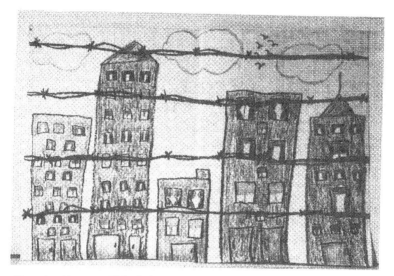

Figure 2.1 Cityscape with barbed wire

and protect it, but also longs to be the source of this perfection. Segal could have been describing the pottery studio. I had observed many patients working with clay. More often than not they responded to the soft, comforting material, molding it into a desired object. It was malleable, flexible and the barrel in which the clay was kept seemed bottomless, inexhaustible. Patients possessed the material, created something new with it and found themselves to be the source of that perfect moment of creation. I had observed the harshest, most hostile of patients almost miraculously grow pliable in attitude while working with clay in their pottery studio.

The art room, however, was a larger room, full of sharp edges, uncooperative materials and memories of teachers who told students they couldn't really draw. I thought Jenny might be responding to the difference in the space and the memories it might evoke.

I could not continue to ignore Jenny's changing behavior for long, however. During one session late in the fall of 1985, Jenny created a soft mound which she smoothed and stroked with water, an activity that clearly resembled symbiotic contentment. Suddenly her mood changed. She wanted a tool to fill the mound with holes, to make a pencil holder. She could not be dissuaded and the mound was attacked with what looked like vicious abandon. At the end of this session Jenny stated with some agitation that she

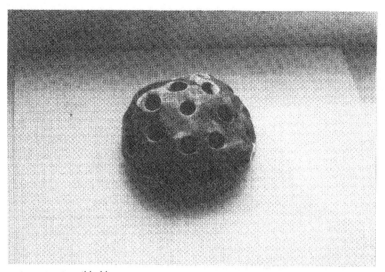

Figure 2.2 Pencil holder

would be seeing her psychiatrist again after the psychiatrist's six-month maternity leave. It would seem Jenny made an association between the breast shape and the therapist who had deprived her for six months. It became vital that she fill the breast full of holes, discharging her rage with a certain amount of regulation and control. It was also vital that she then turn this into something functional, so that the rage could be expressed but transformed into a gift, a pencil holder (Figure 2.2).

The next session with Jenny was in the art room. She seemed to be busy creating and destroying a large black tear. She would almost complete one, destroy it and try another. During this process Jenny stated that her psychiatrist would not be able to see her any more. With some intervention Jenny completed the tear, explaining that she had no feelings at all. She stated that her therapist had told her to trust her, that she would come back after having a baby. 'Why did she have to go and have a dumb old baby, anyway?' As Jenny colored the tear with black crayon and ran barbed wire across the picture, she stated the tear didn't mean anything, that she was just a little sad about life, and she really couldn't cry. At this point I noticed a resemblance between the tear and the clay 'pencil holder', so I said that the tear looked like a lot of 'bad stuff; bad mother stuff or bad psychiatrist stuff'. Jenny responded to this with the association of her first memory of wanting to die, of taking a bottle of aspirin, of being told by her mother that she could stay with the doctor for doing that. She made a further association to a time when she was four and her mother left her on the steps of City Hall, but the courts made the mother take Jenny back. When questioned as to whether or not such memories might not make Jenny a little sad, Jenny responded that the tears she drew belonged to 'Carey', who lived in her body but was thin, pretty and had it all together.

The chart

After this session I went to the chart room to check Jenny's diagnosis and history. (Seeing as many people in a week as we did, I am embarrassed to say charts were only read after something remarkable occurred.) Her chart contained a detailed report from a referring agency and seemed to be material taken from interviews with her. It stated that she was third of seven siblings and had often been beaten by her mother and siblings. This was justified by a story that she had been adopted, a story which she had not questioned until she was 12. Her first suicide attempt was at the age of three, following the death of an uncle. She had seen him lying peacefully with a smile on his face at the funeral. Around this time her mother had told her never to take more than two aspirin or she would be dead like her uncle. Jenny had felt it would be better to be dead than alive and continually beaten by the members of her family. She reported that while in the hospital having her stomach pumped, her mother had tried to get the doctors to keep her.

At the age of six Jenny developed migraines after her father had tried to kill her by choking her. He said he would kill her if she ever talked about it. She also reported having been raped at this time. She began therapy at the age of eight. At this point the chart began to include references to gaps in her memory and activities that she couldn't understand. When her father lay dying in a hospital with cancer of the esophagus, Jenny visited him every day for two years. She didn't know why she felt compelled to visit him, since each visit was so painful. When she was in twelfth grade she began a six-year stretch with a therapist at Bellevue Hospital whom she reported she never said a word to. During the seventh year the therapist left the hospital and Jenny tried to commit suicide. During that period she went to City University of New York and got a BA in sociology, but she had no memory of college at all. Jenny had then worked for the telephone company for three years but was fired for migraines, dizziness and writing numbers backwards. She also worked in a church-run day care center but was fired and brought up on charges of arson and then was acquitted for lack of evidence. She reported a history of, once a month, since her adolescence, stealing things that she didn't want or need. Jenny reported hearing voices of men and women inside her, telling her she was bad. The chart gave her diagnosis as paranoid schizophrenia, but the history of child abuse, migraines, dizziness, periods of amnesia, a childlike personality, concern with choking, suicide attempts and hearing internal voices were all indicators of DID (at that time MPD) (Kluft 1985a). (Jenny's psychiatrist later admitted that the choice of diagnosis was simply the justification for his choice of medication and treatment.)

The treatment

In order to look at Jenny's use of art therapy I will summarize the work that was documented along with her reactions from early spring of 1987 to late spring of 1988 (Gerity 1997). This will provide an overview of how a dissociative individual is able to use art therapy. Hypotheses about the actual agents of change could be inferred from this overview. I had been working with Jenny for a year and a half by the spring of 1987 and had established a positive rapport. She seemed fairly comfortable in both the art room and the pottery studio. She had joined the puppet-making group, where various parts of herself began to emerge more clearly.

Over the years this puppet-making group had various co-leaders, usually drama therapists or interns in drama therapy and art therapy. It was our task to maintain a group that was fluid and flexible enough to allow for the patients to create various characters out of papier mâché and cloth and to then imbue them with story and personality. We were also responsible for keeping clear boundaries and limits, so that the group would be safe from the annihilation urges of a destructive puppet, a representation of an internalized 'bad object'. In order to maintain the balance between fluidity and structure, we would create puppets alongside the patients, neutral puppets or puppets that had some mythic qualities on which the group could project freely. Through these puppets we could encourage imaginative play while maintaining a sense of group structure.

At the beginning of each puppetry group the patients would retrieve their puppets from their little shoe box homes, painted and stacked in one of the bookcases. During the session some members would be working on puppets, creating, fixing or remodeling, while others played and interacted with one another. At the end of each session, the puppets were carefully returned to their little homes. The puppets were treated like very special objects. I'd even

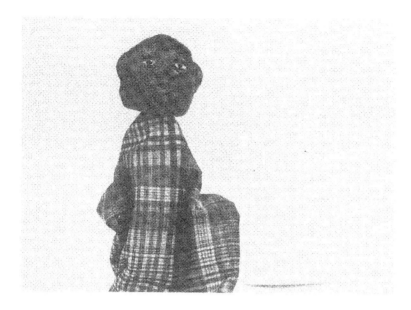

Figure 2.3 Eric

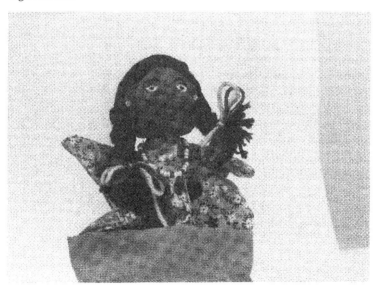

Figure 2.4 Joy

heard the humming of a lullaby upon occasion as the shoe box was put back on its shelf.

The first puppet Jenny created was a male puppet, Eric, a representation of her psychiatrist (Figure 2.3). Eric was extremely wise and thoughtful. Before he spoke there was always a pause, as if he were thinking about how best to phrase his utterances. His wisdom and calm demeanor were admired by all and soon other patients began creating representations of their own wise psychiatrists as well.

The second puppet to be created was Joy, who represented that part of Jenny that was actually being treated at a separate agency (Figure 2.4). This other agency was predominantly a creative arts rehabilitation center and Jenny (or Joy as she was known there) saw two music therapists for individual treatment. This personality-part, Joy, was very childlike, sweet, outgoing and loved to sing. She would appear at our center whenever there was a talent show. The puppet reflected all of these qualities. Perhaps because this puppet and the personality-part it represented seemed to be so easygoing and without problems to work out, or perhaps because Joy was in treatment at another center, we didn't see as much of Joy the puppet as we did the other puppets.

The third puppet created was Carey (Figure 2.5). Carey represented that part of Jenny that was very difficult to be around. She was self-centered, spoke loudly, and didn't care what people thought of her. Her dress was a beautiful patchwork of fiery red and she had little red star earrings. She was as strong and sure of herself as Joy was sweet and self-effacing.

At this point in the puppetmaking we began to see Jenny experimenting and actually becoming more confident in her work. Lisa was created, with a little handkerchief apron and an extremely large baby to take care of (Figures 2.6 and 2.7). Lisa was a representation of Dr Lisa, the psychiatrist who had gone on maternity leave. At the time Jenny made Lisa, she was actually being treated by Eric and awaiting Lisa's return.

Lisa's baby was a puppet at least as big as his mother. He had a fully formed, open mouth and a little bottle. At one point in the group the bottle was seen metaphorically as bad, too small, so I created one out of paper that was three times the size of the puppet, which delighted Jenny no end. The nature of this group made it possible to address these needs and issues through non-threatening metaphor and interactive roleplay. One can imagine the reception one would get in saying to a patient, 'You are very

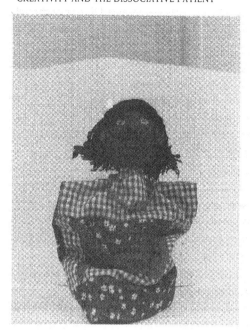

Figure 2.5 Carey

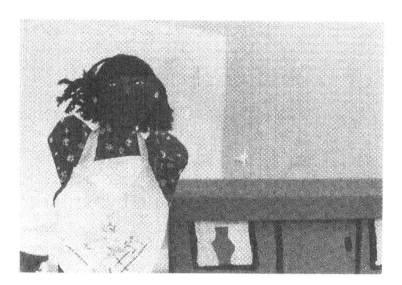

Figure 2.6 Lisa

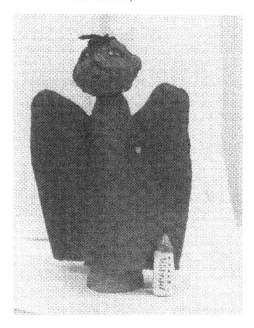

Figure 2.7 Baby

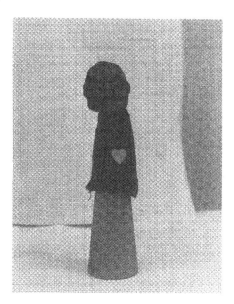

Figure 2.8 Mr Mad

needy and acting like a baby who wants a bigger bottle.' But this was essentially what I was saying in play and it was easily accepted in this form.

A puppet we saw a great deal of was Mr Mad, also fire-engine red (Figure 2.8). This was a very phallic finger puppet, with no arms. He was forever rapping his hard little head on the table in annoyance, giving himself headaches. The other patients delighted in his anger. He so easily expressed some of the things they wished to express but didn't dare. Because he had no arms he was not seen as a real threat to anyone except himself, when he got the urge to rap his head on the table. When asked what he was so mad about he said he didn't really know. One patient pulled out his own psychiatrist/ psychoanalyst puppet and a little wooden analytic couch complete with pillow, and offered his services to Mr Mad to get to the root of his 'madness'. Mr Mad agreed, free associated on the couch and, through possibly the fastest psychoanalysis on record, learned that because he had grown up in a completely mad family, where everyone was mad all the time, that was what he learned to be.

Margaret was seen as very different from Mr Mad (Figure 2.9). She was seen as a very threatening puppet to most of the group members but especially to Jenny. She was a representation of Jenny's mother. She was made with the most care, with tiny carefully painted features, gold earrings, hair that was various shades of gray, and a beautiful blue patchwork dress with a piece of embroidered handkerchief at the center. She, for the most part, stayed hidden in her own shoe box with a jailer or keeper puppet that I had created (Figure 2.10). This puppet, Sebastian, was named by Jenny and given his function by her as well. He was to keep the other puppets safe from Margaret and Margaret safe from them.

Finally, the puppet that Jenny was working on in February of 1987, when I began to document our work together, was Lita, a representation of her counselor at the center (Figure 2.11). Lita had a sweet, open expression on her face and was a good-hearted puppet representing a good-hearted counselor. Around that time Jenny (or Joy) had taken her puppets to the center where Joy received treatment to show one of her music therapists. While explaining to the therapist who each puppet was and who they represented, she realized for the first time that Lisa and Eric looked as though they represented African-American people but in actuality they represented white people, while the puppet representing Lita, a white counselor, looked like a white person. Jenny/Joy was baffled how she never noticed this glaring visual 'mistake'.

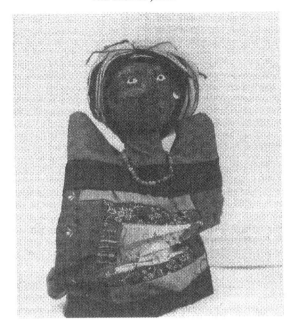

Figure 2.9 Margaret

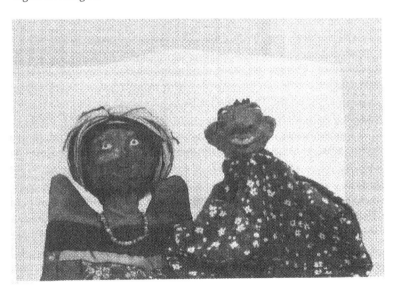

Figure 2.10 Sebastian

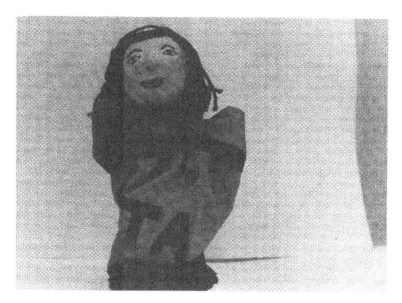

Figure 2.11 Lita

As Jenny became more comfortable in the art room and became more expressive with the puppets, some awareness of object constancy emerged. She spoke of realizing that she didn't have to rush through things to try to get something done all at once, that she could put things away and come back to them. She was beginning to trust that she *could* come back to things. She reflected on the importance of flexibility as well. 'You can't expect things to come out just right. The more flexible you are about how things are going to turn out the more enjoyment you get,' she said (Gerity 1997, p.34).

I noted, though, that Jenny was struggling to understand the idea of having two opposing feelings at the same time, a very difficult concept for the dissociative client who prefers to wall off various feeling states. In the puppetry group she was again using Mr Mad and talking with the drama therapist's depressed blue finger puppet, Hound Dog. Hound Dog explained that the drama therapist was making a new puppet and so he was depressed. Mr Mad suggested that Hound Dog get mad sometimes, that this would give him some energy, to which Hound Dog responded he was all blue and couldn't feel anything except blue. Being the ever-vigilant art therapist, always in search of a visual metaphor, I rooted around in some felt pieces until I found a little red heart, which I quietly brought over to Jenny, not wanting to interrupt the process. Without missing a beat Mr Mad asked Hound Dog if he wanted to feel mad, that if he had a red heart he could feel other things than blue. Hound Dog was pleased with this solution, so Jenny glued the little heart onto the Hound Dog puppet. Then Hound Dog asked Mr Mad if he didn't need a blue heart to feel other things besides mad, to which Mr Mad responded gleefully 'Yes'. Back I trotted to the felt scraps for a little blue heart which I gave to the drama therapist who then glued it onto Mr Mad. Jenny seemed delighted with this interaction, and the drama therapist and I certainly were happy with this acceptance of two distinct feeling states in the one puppet. We saw it as opening the way for learning tolerance of ambivalence.

Later that spring, Jenny and several of the other puppetry group members learned that their counselor was leaving the center. Jenny had just finished her Lita puppet. A discussion ensued about some of the patients feeling silly playing with puppets, feeling like kids. Jenny was looking down at her puppets and she said she took them very seriously. They continued to talk about how sometimes it was very embarrassing to speak through the puppets and to find the puppets saying the most awful things, and that sometimes the puppets spoke more openly and honestly than they were comfortable with. Then the discussion turned to the counselor's leaving. Jenny offered to put Lita, the puppet (representing their counselor), into a large cardboard box painted black with 'City Dump: Home for Bad Puppets' in white letters on the side. This box was created so that a puppeteer could discard a difficult part of herself without destroying the puppet. The patients quickly forgot their resistance to playing with puppets and discussed all the options for visitation rights and which puppet would check on her in the dump on a regular basis. They seemed to be deeply involved in this way of holding onto their beloved counselor and expressing their anger with her as well.

After that session I decided to try interviewing Jenny's puppets outside of the puppetry group. This was a completely novel concept, based on a time-tested qualitative research technique, but with a twist. I was not interviewing the subject directly, but interviewing characters or personalities represented by or projected onto her puppets. We used a tape recorder, and Jenny understood the tapes would be part of the research documentation I was doing at that time.

During this initial interview process Jenny was eager to express a certain level of competence in child rearing. She gave her puppet Lisa advice on how to care for her two-year-old son, the large, needy baby puppet discussed earlier. Her advice was, 'Give him love, give him understanding, and be patient and everything will work itself out.' This advice seemed to be in direct opposition to the way she was raised, to the things she had learned from her own childhood. I recalled Mr Mad's madness being something he had learned from growing up in a completely mad family. During the interview, Mr Mad talked about how having two kinds of feelings was good, but that he might like to feel happy once in a while, that he needed a new heart of a happy color, like yellow.

What started as an attempt to obtain information, interviewing with a tape recorder, met with such success that it evolved into a therapeutic intervention, a staple in our therapeutic relationship. I transcribed our interviews and often gave Jenny excerpts of particularly insightful sessions. This was another way of softening the barriers between feeling states or personality-parts. These interviews were a way to reach an extremely guarded person. This was a window out of which Jenny, Carey and Joy could observe the world and a window through which they allowed me to interact with them. Although it was a way to reach these various parts of her personality, one should keep in mind that Jenny was playing the role of puppeteer. She was identifying with the person who is in control of all the characters. She was allowing me to approach her, and her dissociative identities, in a respectful and serious manner, but because puppets were being used there was also a crucial element of play, of the unexpected, and of possibility for change.

During the summer, while reviewing a log I had been keeping of Jenny's work, I noticed that in the pottery groups Jenny would often approve of something she was working on and then, almost in the next breath, would disapprove and sometimes even destroy her work. After a moment of pride she would express a destructive kind of criticism. I wondered if it was something in her relationship with Margaret, her mother, that caused her to attempt to destroy that thing that made her happy, which I will explore later. By keeping a log, observing behaviors and changes over time, I was able to question Jenny about them either directly or through the metaphors that art provided. An example of this was being able to elicit from Mr Mad a willingness to try yet another feeling and another color of heart to go with it. Subtle changes could be observed, documented and enhanced through this log-keeping process, something that could not necessarily happen with all of the other individuals in groups. Therapists had to keep alert to many things and often subtleties would slip past one.

That summer Jenny began a journal that she kept in my office. Initially she had wanted it to explain more of who she was and how she came to her current life situation. The first entry was written during the entire month of June, without notation of dates, and contained her entire history written in her words. There were many statements full of despair and hopelessness. This journal became an additional source of communication. She could write about her reactions to the things that occurred in art therapy. At one point she wrote that perhaps having her own puppets at home would be of more comfort to her than her stuffed animals, because she had made them after all and they had their own personalities, very real personalities that had taken a lifetime to develop. I believe she was realizing for the first time that she was actually responsible for her own satisfaction. I made note of the idea of her wish to have something at home and was able to put it to good use, which we will see shortly.

In early fall, Jenny's psychiatrist (Eric) talked with Jenny's new counselor and together they decided that Jenny should work with her puppets to bring out more cooperation between Joy and Carey. I was enlisted in this effort and to this end I interviewed the puppets Joy and Carey and attempted to discuss the concept of cooperation. Carey let me know in no uncertain terms that keeping things separate, keeping Joy and Jenny in the dark, was very important to her. She even said she liked to hurt Jenny and Joy, giving Jenny migraines for example. She said, 'I am evil and I like to hate. I see things in black and white' (Gerity 1997, p.38). Although at first glance the session did not appear to go well, because we seemed to be working with Eric's agenda rather than Jenny's, I now got a clearer idea of the internal dynamic between Jenny, Carey and Joy.

That fall Jenny's concerns about her suicidal roommate Sally emerged. Sally was a very big, blonde woman from the Ozark mountains. She and Jenny had met during a hospitalization and they discovered that they shared quite a bit in common; histories of abuse, various 'other people' living inside them and a love of food. They decided that they should room together and save some money, both being dependent on public assistance. They also both received music therapy from the other creative arts center. For a short time Sally attended our center as well, but didn't like the scheduling of so many groups and activities, so she 'let' Jenny have this space for herself. However, being 'allowed' to have one's own space seemed to be a growing problem.

In puppetry Jenny talked about her roommate's threatened suicide. Both the drama therapist and I asked Jenny's psychiatrist puppet about the issue of destructive and dependent relationships between our various puppets. Jenny's psychiatrist puppet spoke eloquently about the need for gradual practicing of independence, that if one puppet leaves for a short period of time and then comes back the other puppet can learn that just because one leaves for a while doesn't mean that one has to leave for ever. Later in the session, Jenny stated she didn't know why but puppetry made her feel better. I pointed out that our puppets' problems were similar to her own situation with her roommate and that the psychiatrist puppet had helped find a solution and that solutions to problems sometimes make people feel better, giving them a sense of inner satisfaction.

A constant refrain in Jenny's journal writing at this time was the suffering and pain of her present situation that she went through in silence. In reading Lister's (1982) article, 'Forced silence: A neglected dimension of trauma', a discussion of the reluctance that a victim has to speak, I was struck by the similarities of the case material and discussion to what was emerging with Jenny: '... the consequences of having been traumatized cannot be ... understood ... outside the context of their prolonged silence after the event. In silence, the pain and subliminal memories of pain festered' (Lister 1982, p.873). This was a constant theme in Jenny's writings. There was an internal pain and anger that was festering and growing out of control. 'If a victim looks for help, or goes further and recounts the trauma, there is a sense that a "promise" has been broken, that retaliation becomes possible or likely or even inevitable' (Lister 1982, p.874). In Jenny's chart there was the reference to years with a therapist spent in silence. She was probably terrified to speak about her history. She sometimes seemed to need to sulk silently in groups, and with Lister's article in mind I would hand her paper and pencil, thinking that the prohibition to keep silence might not include art or writing. Usually the paper and pencil were used to write out the inner dialogues that were troubling her. It certainly seemed to be easier for her to write these dialogues than to talk about them in group.

Her chart described her father's threat that he would kill her if she talked about him and in her writings she expressed threats of pain and domination from Carey if Jenny talked about her. Lister believed that threat, vulnerability, the fear of repetition and a self-protective compliance form fertile ground for learning a masochistic stance. Lister also believed that the child's wish for her parents (or the uninvolved parent) to know, to intuit what has happened, was another precursor to the masochistic stance. The parents' failure to elicit some report of the trauma would then be perceived as an act of hostility (Lister 1982).

Jenny repeatedly let us know that she still had a fantasy that people will know what is happening to her and that something will be done without her having to break her silence, just as she had wished that the school system could have seen her bruises and done something. There were references in her writings about not being able to take much more of the demands of family pressures, but there was no understanding that she would have been safe if she exercised control over these pressures. There was only the passive wish that these pressures would go away, that someone would kill her or that she would die.

Lister believed that this pattern of trauma may begin at an age when some degree of merging with the 'perpetrator' is developmentally normal. To break this bond by speaking of the trauma requires the 'victim' to separate from the 'perpetrator' which may feel like an impossible loss. Rather than accept the loss, the 'victim' will tolerate abuse, remain in physical or psychological 'bondage', and honor the command for silence, remaining close enough to attempt to 'cure' the parent (Lister 1982).

Although Jenny reported hating her mother, she continually tried to please her. Any threat of loss or separation was seen as an attack and usually resulted in Jenny acting out this 'attack' in some way, usually with a somatic complaint. She stated that she felt that her body was leaving her and slowly breaking down. 'To understand these cases and apply what we have learned about trauma in general, we must realize the power of the threat and the tenacity of the victim's psychological relationship with the victimizer' (Lister 1982, p.875). This was not only true for Jenny's relationships with her mother and Sally, but was also true for her internal relationships.

The issue of body image and weight were a central theme that fall. In a puppet interview, Joy admitted Jenny was terrified to lose anything, even a single pound. During this interview Joy described her arrival in Jenny's life, at the age of six when Jenny was raped. She believed Jenny needed to be heavy ever since that time because men would then find her less desirable. Joy wasn't so sure that that was necessary any more.

In the art room these body image concerns were put into her creation of full body image representations in the form of dolls. She had made little papier-mâché heads, hands and feet. She began to cut out little fabric bodies, but had cut one too small. She then had to re-cut it and began free associating to the vulnerability of her pottery and her own body. After expressing these concerns she then successfully created a cloth body that matched the hands, head and feet, as if expressing the concerns and fears was helpful in the resolution of the doll's body. The cloth was now able to connect the separate body parts, making a whole body image representation. This was an exercise in putting together, in making whole, and a very different thing from her journal writings, which were filled with references to internal splitting and attacking of self and body image.

In pottery I pointed out to Jenny that her slab work was related to the creation of dolls, in that she was putting pieces together to create something new and whole, not to mention beautiful and useful. She wrote in her journal about the feeling of control she had when measuring and fitting the slabs together. She also expressed the fact that it took her full attention and created a soothing feeling. She described creating pinch pots as also being a way of slowing down and focusing, watching a form slowly emerge from the clay. Sometimes, however, Carey would step in and destroy a piece. She wrote that Joy would then feel so bad she would feel self-destructive. She felt she had no control over Carey's destructiveness. But the reality was that for her, clay was very therapeutic, either pinching or building with slabs, and she intended to continue working with it even after leaving the center, 'by whatever means possible'.

My thoughts in reading this, I told her, were that everyone had their own role and even Carey had the role of critic and that she didn't need to feel hurt or self-destructive when Carey was critical, since Carey seemed to want everyone to do their very best.

In an effort to understand the helplessness that Jenny and Joy expressed about Carey's destructive urges, I turned to Krystal's (1978) article, 'Trauma and affects', a clear discussion of the feelings of helplessness, the difficulty in verbalizing concerns and the need for somatization of victims of trauma.

Krystal reviewed Freud's concept of trauma, suggesting that the feeling of helplessness was key to understanding why a situation is traumatic. The traumatized individual feels helpless, feels that his or her own strength is inadequate for the situation. This is a reality for children who are being abused. Their strength *is* inadequate to defend themselves.

Krystal pointed out that there was an accompanying inability to verbalize emotions and that these emotions were then expressed in psychosomatic disease such as migraine, ulcer and arthritis. This kind of expression, non-verbal and not a symbolic representation, he considered to be a 'regression in affective expression' (p.95).

We can observe this psychosomatic disease process in Jenny, in her constant quests for treatment of somatic complaints. She had many doctors that she saw at various clinics all over Manhattan. One cardiologist told her she had to lose weight, another doctor told her she was losing too much weight too quickly, and that she would be in a wheelchair for the rest of her life. She saw a specialist for her arthritis, who said she had osteoporosis and would be in a wheelchair for the rest of her life. Another doctor told her that she was producing too much calcium in her joints and that it would have to be removed or she would be in a wheelchair the rest of her life. Of course, this is all her report, but we can read into it a dread and an expectation of returning to that helpless state that Freud referred to. One aspect of her arthritis and migraine was that it often occurred when her mother wanted something from her. Her journals were filled with conflicts over physically not being able to meet her mother's needs.

Krystal also spoke of emotions themselves being 'trauma screens; hence there is a fear of one's emotions and an impairment of affect tolerance' (Krystal 1978, p.98). This explained why Jenny constantly referred to her feelings as being overwhelming and intolerable. After reading this it seemed even more important to point out at every opportunity where Jenny did have control and power.

Later in the fall I announced that I would be attending an art therapy conference for a few days. Jenny seemed to be having difficulty with this and with a few other life crises. I decided to interview Mr Mad (to Jenny's great relief) as this was one puppet who was 'allowed' to express anger without fear of damage or retribution. Mr Mad was able to explain that when Jenny gets mad, she might sabotage things she is working on. She doesn't want to show her anger. Mr Mad focused on how people took advantage of Jenny, how her mother demanded that she shop for her even though her arthritis made it impossible, how Sally got a dog and got her to take out a loan and then on top of all that thought she may be pregnant. Life was too difficult so Jenny was feeling overwhelmed by her feelings, suicidal.

Dr Laurie Wilson, professor at New York University, had observed in a lecture on psychoanalysis of the artist that 'masochism was an attempt to preserve or restore hope through a display of pathos' and I was on the lookout for new ways for Jenny to restore hope. I suggested to Mr Mad that we help Jenny learn to set limits and we help Jenny find some value about herself. Mr Mad thought that both of these ideas were good ones.

Before I actually left for the conference, Jenny came into the art room 'so angry at her counselor' that she didn't know if she would be at the center when I returned. In the middle of this angry tirade she switched and became very young sounding, saying that she would never leave the center as long as I was there. Intuitively responding to this childlike voice, I retrieved a papier-mâché and cloth doll similar to the ones that she was working on and told her that the doll would keep her company while I was away. The doll, Sweet Basil (named by Jenny), was a prop used in the puppetry group so Jenny was very familiar with it and seemed delighted with the suggestion (Figure 2.12). I had remembered from her journal entry in June that she had been feeling lonely and was wishing she'd had her puppets there to talk to. If I was to be away at a conference, she might also wish to have someone to talk to, even possibly a doll I had made, a transitional object for that childlike part of her that couldn't tolerate abandonment. She accepted the doll graciously.

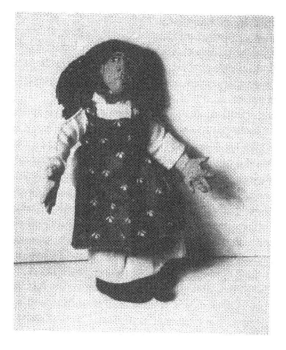

Figure 2.12 Sweet Basil

During the time I was away, she wrote a dialogue between herself and Sweet Basil, written up like a puppet interview transcript. Together they 'discussed' the possibility of setting limits with her mother, that it would really be all right since she wouldn't be doing it out of anger but out of physical concerns for her own health. Sweet Basil sounded rather wise, but unwilling to suggest that Jenny would be entitled to be angry about her mother's treatment of her, past and present.

Once again we have an example of something that began as a simple intervention, something for her to 'hold' while I was away, developing into something much more. Sweet Basil became an internalized good object, a character in Jenny's repertoire of characters and another window through which she could look at the world and through which we could communicate.

Once I got back from the conference Jenny went into overdrive on dollmaking. She worked very carefully, picking out cloth and cutting it. She said it had to be the perfect size in order to match the head, just like the first ones were perfectly matched in size. As she was working on the last head she said she felt that they were getting better and better, a positive evaluation of her own work (Figure 2.13). She had shown her dolls to many people, Eric, her counselor and various staff members, and since everyone wanted one, she decided she would sell them for ten or fifteen dollars a piece depending whether a therapist or a doctor was buying the doll (sliding scale).

After this positive evaluation of her work she brought in pages and pages of her journal writing that were full of helplessness, hopelessness, sadness and confusion. I decided to give her a homework assignment. When she wrote her feelings in her journal and a negative self-destructive feeling came out, she was to follow it with a positive statement, like 'Lani and Sweet Basil really do care about me'. The idea came out of attending Marcia Rosal's presentation at the 1987 American Art Therapy Association conference on cognitive work, training schizophrenics to 'talk to themselves'. My interpretation of the presentation, for Jenny, was this. If you have two statements like a) I feel hopeless, and b) So-and-so likes me a whole lot, then they are both true statements. But you feel very differently if you say 'So-and-so likes me, but I feel hopeless' as compared with 'I feel hopeless, but so-and-so likes me'. This made sense to Jenny and she employed the homework assignment with great success.

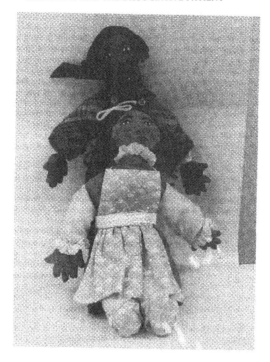

Figure 2.13 Dolls

Later in the month she wanted to give me two dolls. I suggested we trade a drawing of mine that she particularly liked for the two dolls. The drawing was of an old man and a little boy and it was carefully drawn in pencil with various shadings and tones. In an interview with Carey we discussed the drawing. Carey had been describing Jenny's inability to see the shades of gray in life: 'Jenny doesn't know anything but black and white. Things are either this way or that. There is nothing in between.' I pointed out to Carey that Jenny liked the drawing of the old man and boy and that the drawing was nothing *but* shades of gray. There was no black and white in it. Out of this discussion Carey came up with a title for the drawing: 'There is beauty in shades of gray.'

In an art group in December Jenny had dolls' body parts spread out in front of her. She showed others in the group her progress, pointing out which one needed hands, which needed a new head since she had thrown one away. She talked about various techniques in stuffing and sewing the bodies and how she was trying to make the bodies more uniform. She counted all the heads, hands and feet and then stated several times that the hands were the hardest to do. This activity of counting, matching and discussing technique seemed to give Jenny pleasure.

Her journal entries began to focus on a man who worked in a restaurant on Madison Avenue. His name was Ralph and it seemed Jenny was quite taken with him. He would offer her pieces of cake, or if she seemed to be dieting, pieces of melon. Ralph seemed to be a very thoughtful man. Her journal entries also expressed her feeling of aggression turned against herself:

> I gained 4lb. And I feel like cutting my body into pieces and throwing away the parts in different directions because I don't care about myself anymore. Oh, I forgot something. Lani and Sweet Basil care about me a whole, whole lot and that makes me feel better. (Gerity 1997, p.47)

In an interview with the puppet Joy, the discussion turned to Jenny's feelings about Ralph, her interest in exploring the possibility of a relationship, but also the confusion and fear and mistrust of his intention. I let her know that feelings and memories from the past sometimes affect us today. They may have been stuffed into a closet for a long time and need to come out slowly in a very safe place where they can be sorted through and talked about. Joy then described the event that had marked her arrival, Jenny's rape by a 16-year-old neighbor when she was only six. She then began to weep. I let her weep and patted Joy on the back (Jenny's hand). Finally the discussion continued and moved back to Ralph. Both Joy and I decided that Jenny was grown up now and didn't have to do anything she didn't want to do.

Towards the end of the month she learned that her unit supervisor was leaving, which began to elicit familiar abandonment concerns and a great deal of negative feelings about her own self-worth. She was not aware that her counselor was soon to follow, due to office politics and administrative hostility, things I was aware of. Concerned with the repercussions of her learning about this further abandonment, I again reminded her that the things that happen to us in the past affect our lives today. I suggested that she was taught to believe some very negative things about herself. I then asked her if she would consider thinking about how she could learn new things and think about some goals she might like for the future.

In reviewing all of the interviews, journal entries and notes I had collected, to that point, one of Jenny's statements stood out:

I think I have and had so many headaches because I had to hold so much in and I was not allowed to express myself. My mother used to tell me don't speak until you're spoken to so I never spoke. I stayed silent. I said nothing and I felt nothing. (Gerity 1997, p.48)

Within this statement I saw the core of Jenny's difficulties as well as the basis for goals of her treatment. She described an inability to express herself as causing her somatic pain. She stated that her mother told her not to speak and she described her willingness to comply. There was an edge to this statement that hinted at the anger Jenny felt toward her mother. But she could not trust her feelings, so she said nothing and she felt nothing.

My thinking was that if Jenny were to feel safe within our relationship she might be able to begin to symbolize her feelings in a variety of ways rather than exclusively somatically, to feel free to speak and to comply only when she wished, whether with Ralph or with her mother, and most of all I hoped that Jenny would feel comfortable with her feelings towards herself and others.

Throughout the material reviewed there had been repeated descriptions of trauma both in the past and present. Things that were done to her in the past were repeated over and over. She sought out relationships that re-enacted and confirmed her past. If these relationships weren't harsh enough she was able to create internal dramas that reflected her early traumas. In the past Jenny was bound in a masochistic relationship with her mother and other family members. These relationships persisted. She also found a roommate who fulfilled this role for her. Within her fragmented internal world she assigned various roles for Carey, Joy and Jenny. Carey often took the role of the punitive super ego or sadistic mother, while Jenny played the role of the helpless child. Joy remained on the outside of this relationship and seemed able to function despite the struggles that occurred.

T. H. Ogden (1986) provided a theoretical matrix with which to understand what Jenny may have been going through in the material found in these notes, journals and transcripts. Ogden discussed the 'object-component' as the patient's ego sub-organization which is identified with the mother; in Jenny's case this would be Carey who is most like Margaret and is seen in relation to the self-component or the self. He described how the object-component (Carey) may feel envious of the self (Jenny) for enhanced feelings of self-esteem.

Ogden wrote that the internal object relationship consisted of a mutually dependent mother–child relationship in which the child was willing and eager to be masochistic if that would help bind her to the sadistic mother who was felt to be always on the verge of abandoning her. He felt that the nature of this ultimate threat is replicated internally with the threats from the object-component to abandon the self-component.

The object-component, in this case Carey, wished to sap feelings of well-being from its object, Jenny, and make those feelings of well-being its own. Ogden felt it was important for the object-component to maintain connectedness with, or control over, the self-component. Signs of increasing independence on the part of the self-component will be enviously attacked if the object-component begins to fear change or of being left behind (Ogden 1986, pp.161–163).

Searles (1979) also vividly described clinical data in which the patient unconsciously functioned as multiple people, one of whom may become jealous of the other.

Throughout the material I had collected since the spring, there were various examples of this conflict between the object sub-organization of the ego (its various forms being the puppet Margaret, the personality and puppet Carey and the roommate Sally) and the self-component, Jenny. Jenny took a masochistic stance with the sadistic, controlling and jealous object-components, whoever they happened to be at that moment. In her journal writing of June, Jenny expressed the conflict with her mother. 'Every time I think of how my mother beat me up it makes me angry. She was so mean to me but I'm the only one that she can depend on these days … I do things for her to try to please her and she just doesn't appreciate me' (Gerity 1997, p.50). On 17 November, Jenny described Carey's feelings of not wanting anyone to give Jenny any attention. Carey believed that her attention to Jenny was all Jenny needed. She became jealous when others paid attention to her (as in complimenting her pottery or dolls) and would then punish Jenny in various ways. Jenny's relationship to her roommate, Sally, was a constant drama full of guilt, control, threats of suicide and acting out. It seemed that Sally would go to great lengths to keep Jenny in this masochistic position or Jenny would go to great lengths to keep Sally in the dominant, sadistic position. Throughout the material I noticed a recurrent theme of a wish to be saved by a 'good, symbiotic mother' who wouldn't need to be told what's wrong, their connection would be so strong. She would have known that Jenny wanted to wear pants so that boys wouldn't pull up her skirts. Her 'good, symbiotic mother' would have known that Jenny was raped by a neighbor and that her uncle was sexually abusing her. Her school would have done something when they saw her continually bruised and battered. Jenny continually wished to be saved and was continually disappointed. This continual disappointment further confirms Jenny's negative self-image. Lister (1982) described this phenomenon as a wish for the parent to intuit what was going on and if they didn't somehow elicit a report of the trauma the patient would perceive this as an act of hostility. Jenny perceived the failure of an other to intervene in her various crisis situations as not only an act of hostility but a further abuse and confirmation that she was not worth helping. I suspected the continuous emergencies in Jenny's life were not only created out of habit but that they further served as a test for those around her, to see if that good symbiotic mother would ever come for her. After reading several journal entries that described both the mother and Sally as being extremely demanding and abusive, somehow getting Jenny to give them money that she doesn't have, I verbalized to Jenny the unspoken wish that things could be better without having to say anything. I stated that sometimes a knight in shining armor would be nice, but that in reality having things come out all right takes a lot of work. Jenny had smiled at this.

In reviewing the material I saw my first goal as establishing a good working relationship with all of Jenny, especially the more punitive, harsh object-component that Carey embodied. This seemed to be of primary importance after working with another DID patient who was instructed by her therapist not to reveal her destructive aspects. The result was fatal in that case, so it seemed particularly important that I communicate with Jenny's more destructive aspects at the outset and let it be known that I was extremely concerned for her as a whole person. This took some time and was not without setbacks, but Jenny assured me that Carey finally trusted me.

Another goal that I held somewhere in the back of my mind was to provide through artwork an experience that would serve to help Jenny with an integration of her body image. It seemed to me that the various traumas which she had suffered as a child had a great deal to do with a very negative body image and associations of pain and suffering with physical contact. Since the spring, I consciously tried to take every opportunity to reinforce a more positive sense of physical self. Although she continued at times to have dreams that she was in pieces or falling apart, I thought this was being successfully countered by her working very hard to create whole body image representations in the form of dolls. Having found a market and a demand for these dolls, she gave herself the opportunity to create many, many dolls. It seemed that she was soothed and calmed by working on her dolls or working with clay slabs – in both cases putting pieces together to form a whole.

A further and related task or goal at the back of my mind was to help Jenny tolerate affect. It seemed that if she were able to tolerate affect, she would be able to represent it more easily and in less self-destructive ways, as in her preoccupation with various diseases. Krystal (1978) stated that psychosomatic diseases 'represent a regression in affect expression consisting of affect dedifferentiation, deverbalization, and resomatization' (Krystal 1978, p.95). After a session where Jenny seemed to feel safe enough to re-experience a traumatic situation and to weep over the experience, she stated about herself, 'She has so many feelings. She used to not have any feelings at all. Now she has feelings' (Gerity 1997, p.52). This was a continuing battle for Jenny, to try to help her tolerate her feelings. In rereading the material there seemed to be a positive trend in that direction.

Finally it seemed vital that Jenny internalize some positive experiences and attitudes towards herself. One of the most successful interventions in that regard was to suggest that for every negative thing she wrote about herself that she also write the sentence, 'Lani and Sweet Basil care a whole lot.' This was repeated often in her journal. Also providing the transitional object, Sweet Basil, whenever I was away from the center for any length of time seemed to reinforce this positive internalization.

At the end of December Jenny discovered that she would have to lose another counselor. She was very concerned whether or not I liked her. She seemed quite happy when I assured her that I liked her new counselor and that she had her office on my floor and that I knew her quite well. Jenny was not thinking of going into the hospital, which she had done the last time she had lost a counselor.

Our last meeting of the month and year was just before a Christmas break. I wondered how she would be during this break, because of the transition in counselors, so I asked what Sweet Basil might do if she got too lonesome for me, thinking Jenny might more easily speak of Sweet Basil's feelings than her own. Jenny assured me that Sweet Basil would be just fine and that she would take very good care of her.

January was a very difficult month. Jenny made it very clear she was never going to trust anyone ever again: 'They just leave you.' She decided to end her monthly phone contact with Dr Lisa (the psychiatrist that was represented by the puppet, Lisa). This seemed rather drastic, since she had had this phone contact since Dr Lisa had gone on maternity leave more than two years previously. It seemed related to her perceived abandonment by the counselor who had just left, that Jenny was 'identifying with the aggressor' and leaving others.

Several times Jenny came into the art room and drew portraits of strong, angry-looking men, identifying herself as Carey. Her behavior was erratic and she complained of voices and nightmares: 'I had a dream about little kids ripping my body apart and chewing the pieces.' She expressed fear of her new counselor, and not wanting to talk to one of her two music therapists from the other center, Eric or even Sally. She had a panic attack at our center one afternoon when she was sure I had left her. The new counselor came out into the hall where Jenny was weeping and gave her some paper to write her feelings on until the counselor was free to meet with her. This helped the panic attack, but the general aggression which focused towards Jenny from within continued. Carey wrote:

> I will try my best to keep her confused and upset because I can deal better with myself when she is in a state of confusion. I really hate Jenny. If she wants to kill herself she should have a right to. It's her life and nobody else's. (Gerity 1997, p.54)

It seemed this relentless aggression must have had something to do with the abandonment by the previous counselor. I attempted an interview with Mr Mad and Carey to see if something might emerge around the issue of the counselor. These two puppets informed me that the reason the counselor had left was because Jenny was too needy. I decided to explain to them that Jenny's counselor had left because the school she was attending wanted her to have a social work supervisor but that the agency had assigned her to some other kind of supervisor. The school had found a different placement for her. She was *really* sad to leave Jenny but she had to continue her education. The discussion then turned to books which had been difficult to read all the way through, which Jenny had almost not finished, like *The Color Purple*, but of which she had turned the next page and read the next chapter. I suggested that Jenny might remember that when she felt bad, it was a new chapter of her life to explore. We ended the interview with a further discussion about needing to see the shades of gray in things. Carey admitted, in confidence, that it wasn't just Jenny who had difficulty with all of this but that she did as well.

Later in the month Jenny described a dream where she flew with a dragon past clouds and a rainbow. They found Jenny's great-grandmother who was rocking and working on a patchwork quilt for Jenny. What followed this was great resentment that her mother, Margaret, who knew how to make quilts, would not make one for Jenny.

In an interview with Joy we talked about the similarities between Carey and Margaret; how Margaret never showed her children affection and how now it's hard for Jenny to, and how the negative feelings were easier for Margaret to express and now they are the feelings that Jenny is most comfortable with. I suggested that Jenny needed to keep some positive feelings inside her heart even if they were scarier and could go away at any moment:

> …it's important to keep some of that positive stuff in your heart. You can remember the positive stuff so that even if people go away you can remember those things. Like keeping them in a box. That's what hearts are for, I think. If people go away you can keep part of them. (Gerity 1997, p.55)

At the end of the month Jenny gave me a dialogue she had written between Jenny and Sweet Basil, of which the last lines were:

Sweet Basil: I don't like to see you give yourself such a hard time about living. For the moment you are doing your best.

Me: But I'm not doing my best. I hate myself.

Sweet Basil: But I care about you.

Me: I know you do and I appreciate it because there's not very many more people that care about me. You know something Sweet Basil, you make me feel good inside and it's a feeling I'm not used to, so it's a little uncomfortable, but I hope one day I will get used to it and enjoy it. (Gerity 1997, p.56)

During February Jenny continued to express somatic concerns and, in addition to osteoporosis and arthritis, discovered that she had too much calcium in her bones. She would need surgery in June to remove some, and needed to lose weight in order to prepare for this. She was sure that they would cut her legs off and she would be in a wheelchair for the rest of her life.

What was at the back of my mind was the idea that Jenny's mother had not been able to provide her children with enough positive things to nurture them. In an interview with Carey I asked how she felt about positive feelings. She said they made her heart feel like it would fly out of her chest and splatter on the wall. During the interview it came to me that if Jenny created dolls that represented the parts of herself when she was young, she would be able to offer them some of the positive feelings that Margaret had not shown her. I asked Carey if she thought that Jenny might want to create such dolls. Jenny put Carey down and became very enthusiastic and excited about the prospect of making a young Jenny, Carey and Joy. I suggested that we might make a nice safe house for them to live in and that she could make them patchwork blankets. She became very happy about that idea. Later I thought that perhaps patchwork was so important to her because it is an elegant integration of many fragments, a wonderful metaphor for the integration of aspects of the self. During the puppetry group that followed she was able to articulate exquisitely for another patient that 'sometimes you feel guilty for how your puppet can express feelings so easily that you can hardly admit to yourself that you have', sentiments reminiscent of a discussion that had occurred in puppetry in April the year before.

The journal writings continued to include Jenny's fears and aggression. She wrote about having bad thoughts, that she wanted to blow her brains out and take her family with her. At this time I had been reading Shapiro (1988). She quotes Angyal (1982): 'When his neurosis is threatened the person feels that everything is falling to pieces, that he is about to dive into nothing, that he is dying. Parting with neurosis feels like parting with life' (Shapiro 1988, p.9). This certainly fitted Jenny's journal descriptions of her experiences that month. After every positive step there would be a retreat into fear and dissolution. In her journals, Jenny wrote that Sweet Basil told her:

> I can be supportive and not criticize you because you have bad thoughts. Lani can help you too, because she will listen to you or read whatever thoughts you have and give you feedback that will not harm you but make you feel stronger and better about yourself. (Gerity 1997, p.57)

This positive statement filled with her own inner strength, though attributed to Sweet Basil and myself, was followed by a reported trip to see Eric where she told him she felt she was dying, being eaten from the inside by cancer, that she felt separated and scattered in many directions and was afraid to be alone, was afraid that Sally's dog would attack her in the night. She reported that Eric blandly expressed concern that there was always something new wrong with her body.

Towards the middle of the month, Jenny wrote a beautiful description of the beach in South Hampton, followed by concerns of destruction, dying and falling apart, which was then followed by a bit of wisdom from Sweet Basil:

I learned so much from Sweet Basil. She gave me encouragement and a sense of hope. I learned a lot about my attitude about life and death and she said I deserve more respect from myself and she said I should do one really nice thing for myself each week and that I should learn to trust more, but I told her I already know these things but I just get caught up in the blacks and whites and don't think about the shades of gray in my life. (Gerity 1997, pp.57–58)

In art therapy Jenny was finishing up the representations of her various parts as children. Little Joy was finished first. The interview with Little Joy was a review of her childhood traumas. Towards the end of this interview, she switched into the present and told a joke about Sally and her dog. She said:

Sally was in the elevator with Rusty and she said 'sit down honey' and this man sat down in the elevator. His wife said why and he said the lady said sit down honey so I sat down and everyone laughed all the way down 24 floors. (Gerity 1997, p.58)

Such a light-hearted story, especially one about Sally, was very unusual. Perhaps the need to keep Sally in the role of the aggressor was lessening a bit.

This interview was followed by a journal entry of a dialogue between Carey and Sweet Basil. In the journal Carey was enraged with Jenny, she said that she should kill herself and that Carey would help. Then Jenny wrote:

I don't want to face the day anymore. I feel it's not worth feeling so bad. But sometimes I try to think about happy things. The things that make me feel good are coming to the center and especially seeing you and a few other people, also talking to my grandmother, spending money, going for coffee, seeing a child's smile, not aching, working with pottery makes me happier than you can imagine. It makes me forget all my troubles and it soothes me and makes me feel free. I wish I could work with clay more. Also lately in pottery Carey has been helping me appreciate my work more. She's been giving me a positive outlook on what the final product is. I'm not so negative about the finished piece anymore. When I go to the other center and sing I feel good. When I talk to Sweet Basil I feel very trusting and free to express my feelings. I dream about Sweet Basil and she becomes a human and she is very wise in my dreams and she protects me in my dreams now from the monsters and giants that are trying to attack me. She went on a long trip with Rutherford [the flying dragon from an earlier dream] and me to see my great grandmother up high above the clouds and my great grandmother really likes her a lot. She told me to listen carefully to what Sweet Basil had to tell me because she was a real wise and honest person. My great grandmother told me to attempt to make a quilt for my dolls and she will guide me along. She said that it's very important for me to make the quilt because it means so much to me and after I complete it I will be very happy and satisfied and won't need the quilt that my mother promised to make me years ago. Sweet Basil said that my mother making me a quilt will probably never happen and I am wasting energy hoping for something that may never happen. (Gerity 1997, pp.58–59)

Reading this was reassuring in that it seemed that Jenny was internalizing some positive feelings and able to recreate comforting scenes and imagery for herself. Later Jenny came to an art group and worked on her dolls. She had asked me for help with Little Jenny, gluing the head and hands to the body. She had made the separate parts and although perfectly capable of putting the pieces together herself, having done it so many times before, she wanted me to glue them together. Feeling that this was symbolic for her of something positive, I complied. When she saw this doll, she was delighted. She felt it was the most beautiful of the three. She worked on finishing Little Carey as I painted the box that would be their home. She picked out the colors for the outside and the fabric that would be wallpaper.

At the end of the month I interviewed all three dolls (Figure 2.14), the 'kids', and there was much discussion about quilts. Jenny decided that if she could make Margaret's dress, she could make a quilt for the 'kids' and a quilt for Sweet Basil. She felt that she could remember the quilts her great-grandmother had made and that, along with her dream of the great-grandmother's encouragement, would help her. The interview continued and was very different from the interview with Joy. That had been all about trauma and this interview was about how many bad things she had done as a child, describing each act of aggression in detail. She believed Little Carey had developed a mean personality the day that Jenny had decided that she wanted a birthday cake, never having had one before, and made one with too much salt. It was inedible, disgusting to look at and her family laughed at her attempt. This made Little Carey mean.

March's first journal entry began with a decision never to eat again. Jenny felt she had gained too much weight. Then she began to discuss feeling abandoned and depressed because she had spoken with Dr Lisa for the last time. Sweet Basil then reminded Jenny that she and I would be there for Jenny, to which Jenny responded, 'Sweet Basil, you make me feel so human.'

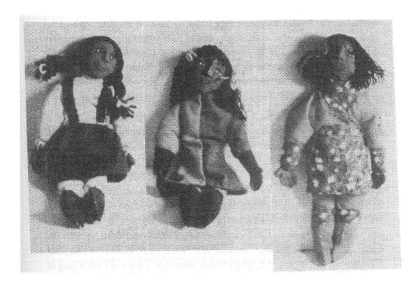

Figure 2.14 Self-representations as dolls (Little Carey, Little Jenny and Little Joy)

In art she began working on a quilt with excitement and in pottery she seemed delighted with her pieces. Interestingly, she did not feel compelled to counter this positive self-regard with anything negative.

During an interview, Little Joy read a book to the others, in which a little boy is afraid of the dark. He is afraid that *something* is going to crawl through the window. His mother gave him some clay and eventually he made a statue of the *something*. He talked to it and wasn't afraid of it anymore. Little Carey expressed envy over Little Joy's ability to read. The discussion then turned to food or the lack of it and the problem of weight. She said, 'I'm always hungry, something is missing in my life'. She thought maybe it was not being wanted or needed by her mom. I suggested that we could let the dolls know they are here because we want them and they could let each other know. Little Carey very bravely said to Little Jenny, 'You know you're here because you're special and I want you to be here ... and even though I haven't known you for very long I still like you and I hope you stay around for a long, long time.' Little Carey then wondered why it was easier to keep those bad feelings inside than it was for the good ones. She said:

It's easier to think about bad things, it's easier to worry about bad things, it's easier to be mad ... but it's very hard to hold on to the positive things and good feelings, and have them and feel them. I wonder why that is? I know Jenny feels so bad for gaining all that weight. And now she's punishing herself and that's so stupid. She feels she has to do something. (Gerity 1997, p.60)

When I asked what that meant Little Carey said: 'Maybe she doesn't have to punish herself. If you think about it, life isn't really that bad.' I replied: 'Well there are some mighty horrible things but there are some mighty good things too.'

Jenny's next journal entry was about her relationship with Sally. Eric, apparently, had wanted Jenny to explore her feelings about Sally because he felt maybe there was something destructive in their relationship. Sally made Jenny feel guilty about coming to the center when she was ill. The problem was that Sally was always ill. Jenny then wished she were dead because she really hated herself. She felt confused and that no one understood her, but then she reminded herself through Sweet Basil that 'Lani and I are trying to understand and to get the three of you to become one and not be so confused and helpless'. After reading this I asked Jenny if change was an easy thing for her to accept. She said no, so I suggested that maybe change was hard for Sally, too. Even little changes like growing independence might make Sally uncomfortable. Jenny nodded.

Finally the 'kids'' quilt was done in time for an interview. They expressed feeling nervous. I asked what makes children nervous. Little Joy replied:

Being frightened, not being sure if your mother is going to send you away or not. When I was five years old my mother took us all to the court house on 163rd street and told us to sit on the steps there until someone came because she could no longer take care of us. Because she didn't have any money to feed us, so we sat there in the hot sun, sweating and crying. And the cops came. We told them that our mother told us to sit there because she couldn't take care of us anymore. They took us inside and gave us water and called our mother and made her come back and get us. They told her she couldn't do that or she would go to jail. (Gerity 1997, p.61)

Then Little Joy continued talking, describing her uncle's sexual abuse of her and her father's attempt to kill her. 'I felt I was all alone,' she said. At the very end of the interview she told, all in a rush, of how as a first-grader there had been a man near her school who had paid her a quarter to let him perform oral sex. The quarter made her feel powerful and she would buy herself ice cream.

Later on in the month Jenny showed me her newest patchwork quilt, the one for Sweet Basil, explaining how it was much nicer than the first, that the pieces were much smaller and the design more beautiful. She expressed pride in her work. Then she began to describe Sweet Basil as being very wise and sweet although maybe a little homely. She described her arms as being ready to accept all the kids in the world. We began to discuss who should be interviewed when Jenny interrupted to blow her nose, complaining of the weather causing a cold or flu. I suggested that she could make herself a big quilt, a comforter for herself, to which she replied that it was very hard to make them. She then said she would make some for the dolls she had made for her nieces, and that her mother would be shocked and would ask who made them. She then said it would be too 'overpowering' to make a big one. That would be too scary. The discussion of making her own quilt seemed to be very important. If Jenny were to show her mother that she could make her own blanket then the mother would never make one for her. As long as she didn't have a blanket there would always be the hope that the mother would one day provide it for her. If Jenny were to care about herself she might somehow lose all hope of getting her mother finally to care for her.

During the last week of March, Jenny learned that a music therapist she had been working with for six years would be leaving the other center. After some discussion Jenny decided that she would make a statue of him as a going-away gift. She began working on a full human figure in clay. If she was able to create a representation of him in clay it would mean that she had internalized him and perhaps would not have as difficult a time with this loss as she had with the last therapist's sudden departure. On the Friday of that week we conducted a very playful interview and discussed what she would do during the time I would be out. We discussed various options. At the end of the interview she took charge of arranging the dolls on the quilt in their box, in a way that they 'would keep each other company and not get into any fights'.

In mid-April, we had an interview which centered around Jenny's loss and abandonment issues. The following is an excerpt:

Lani: I wonder if I can make a little guess about one thing that might be preoccupying you. Let me think. Today is someone's last day here at the center.

Jenny: Who?

Lani: The drama therapist.

Jenny: Oh yeah, I forgot.

Lani: I thought that you might be a little preoccupied with that and that would make you think about the music therapist's leaving the other center.

Jenny: Oh God!

Lani: (*talking to the dolls*) Now I don't know if you guys know this or not, this is something Sweet Basil told me, but that when someone leaves, sometimes Jenny feels it's her fault. And that makes it very hard. It makes it very painful.

Jenny: Yeah.

Lani: So she might not want to think about it because it's such a painful thing. I've experienced this with Jenny before. She'll lock it up or try to lock it up behind a door some place and then she gets headaches or worse, she starts to feel so terrible that she wants to go to the hospital. I'm just really concerned that she's going to feel so bad that she wants to go to the hospital. I'd hate to see her feel so bad. What do you think?

Jenny: (*speaking through Little Jenny*) Well, she's made up her mind that she's not going to the hospital. She has plans for the summer so she has to be really strong and talk about her feelings because that makes her feel better. So when she sees the drama therapist, she'll remember that he's leaving to further his education and not because of her. When she sees the music therapist, well, she can't talk to him yet, she just says let's sing. So he doesn't know how she really feels about him.

Lani: I'll bet she could write him a poem.

Jenny: (*Little Jenny*) That's a good idea. I bet she could.

Lani: (*remembering the sculpture Jenny had been working on of the music therapist*) Where's the sculpture?

Jenny: (*Little Jenny*) Uh oh.

Lani: What do you mean uh oh? Where is the sculpture?

Jenny: (*Little Jenny*) I can't tell you. Carey will tell you.

Lani: Carey wrecked it?

Jenny:	(*Little Jenny*) Carey came in yesterday and she was so mad…
Lani:	Seriously? She wrecked it?
Jenny:	(*Little Jenny*) She did. I tried to stop her but I had no control over her.
Lani:	And I wasn't there to help either.
Jenny:	(*Little Jenny*) You were out. Carey was glad you were out too, because you would have said 'it's all right, it can be fixed' but it fell apart and Carey got so mad she rolled it all together and put it back in the bin and sprinkled water on it and in the afternoon someone used it.
Lani:	Hmmm. I wonder if maybe it could be made again but a little smaller.
Jenny:	(*Little Jenny*) You know Jenny tried and it worked. She got so scared of it that Carey destroyed it. She'll try again today.
Lani:	And maybe a small one this time. I'll bet the size of it made it keep falling apart.
Jenny:	(*Little Jenny*) I know she can do it. I just know she can.
Lani:	Of course. Because we saw the big sculpture.
Jenny:	(*Little Jenny*) That's right. Carey was a brat yesterday. She didn't want to eat the stuff on the diet but she did anyway. One day down.
Lani:	It sounds like Carey needs to talk in puppetry. It sounds like she has a lot of feelings that she needs to take out and look at.
Jenny:	(*Little Jenny*) Yeah, she can't just go around destroying stuff. That's not right.
Lani:	Especially good stuff. It's not like something that just Carey had made, Jenny had worked really hard on it and I even helped make the bench. Carey shouldn't have done that.
Jenny:	(*Little Jenny*) She shouldn't have destroyed the bench. She tried to put the bench back together but she said what's the sense in a bench without anyone to sit on it, so she destroyed that too.
Lani:	Oh, she was real mad.
Jenny:	(*Little Jenny*) Yeah, she had fun doing it too. She said ah-hah, Lani's not here. I'm going to destroy this. She was so devilish yesterday.

Lani:	Is there anything else you want to talk about, besides tattling on Carey?
Jenny:	(*laughing*) Well, I was thinking about my diet. I felt so full yesterday.
Lani:	What were you full of?
Jenny:	Food, the Essex Plan food. Mostly fiber.
Lani:	Great. It's good for you. What about your heart? Does it feel full or empty?
Jenny:	Deprived. But I don't know why. When the food is so delicious why should you feel deprived? That's stupid.
Lani:	Maybe feeling deprived has more to do with getting your emotional needs met. Which maybe when you were little you didn't get. But now we're trying really, really hard. All of us are trying, right?
Jenny:	Yeah, I think I'm trying and Carey and Joy are trying.
Lani:	And Sweet Basil and I try, too. And you've got all your friends here in this nice place. (Gerity 1997, pp.63–64).

The session ended here. It was gratifying to see that it was possible to deal with separation and loss, destruction and reparation.

On 29 April, 1988, we conducted an interview in which Carey talked about the importance of clay. The reclamation of the statue of the music therapist was going well and Carey was cooperating with the others. The following is an excerpt and the final interview to be included in this chapter. We had been discussing Jenny's fire-setting habits as a child.

Lani:	Well, sometimes when little kids have feelings, angry feelings mostly, they look for fires to start, but once they grow up what do they do with their angry feelings?
Carey:	They keep them inside. They don't hurt anyone with them, except themselves.
Lani:	I wonder if there might be some other way to let those feelings out without hurting other people and without hurting yourself.
Carey:	I think it's possible. One way that Jenny lets some of those feelings out is with clay. She may be very soothing and gentle with it, and she has so many feelings inside of her that she wants to create something and all those feelings finally come

out when she finally does. And that helps release some of the angry feelings. If she could really pound the clay and beat the hell out of it, it might make her feel a little better, because she's really restraining herself when she creates something, but feelings still get out anyway and that's the most important thing in her life right now, working with clay. And she's going to the 'Y' again so she can do more with clay since the center won't let her have more pottery groups. Pottery is a very important part of her life. And she needs to be around it and use it as much as possible. I don't know if that makes sense.

Lani: Yes it does.

Carey: It makes sense to her that her angry feelings are lessened when she plays with clay. I don't know, does that make sense?

Lani: It makes sense to me. That's why I studied art therapy. It makes a lot of sense.

Carey: Well, that's how Jenny feels. The more she's around clay the less angry feelings she has and the less depression she has. Today when she works with clay, I'm going to tell her don't think about dying. Think about creating and maybe she'll feel better. I'm going to have a serious talk with her.

Lani: That sounds like a good idea. Part of working with clay, part of the good thing about clay is that it feels soft and nice to work with physically. It just feels good to mush around with the clay. Maybe when you guys were growing up you didn't have so many good physical kinds of feelings. So now you get a chance to work with things that feel good. Also if you bust up something you can make it again.

Carey: Yeah, that's true, but if you bust up something you feel so bad about it. It just feels so bad and it feels like it can't be made again. It's important not to bust it up.

Lani: It is important not to bust it up but sometimes you can't help it.

Carey: I know. Sometimes I just can't stand it when Jenny's having a good time. I just can't stand it. It just gets to me.

Lani: Maybe you could find that it's good for you. Things that are therapeutic for you, not just Jenny. Things that you could enjoy. I think we should find creative ways of expressing ourselves. Don't you think?

Carey: Yeah, I think so. That would help. It would help me leave Jenny's stuff alone. I'm thinking of writing the autobiography. But it's hard. I'm trying to think about my earliest memories. I remember being in a bar with my father, drinking beer with a straw. That's my earliest memory. (Gerity 1997, pp.65–66)

In the chapter that follows we will examine more fully the theories of dissociation, body image and object relations, and then will examine Jenny's history in light of these theories.

CHAPTER 3

Object Relations Theories
and Application

Dissociation

Having access to her artwork, her journal writings, notes from the group and interviews with her gives a fairly clear picture of Jenny's internal world as well as her experience of her external world. This experience seemed filled with aggression, walls and horror, but also with little spaces of respite and creativity. It seemed that most of these spaces, though, were under siege, constantly being battered from within by Carey or by Jenny's own somatic complaints, or from without by Sally or Jenny's mother, Margaret. Often Jenny seemed to call up Sally and Margaret's words just when she was beginning to create something positive for herself. It seemed difficult for her to accept positive experiences and thoughts, and yet the negative experiences and thoughts seemed to drive her to the brink of suicide.

The life Jenny was living was, by her own report, intolerable. She, with her roommate, Sally, seemed to live with the constant shadows of debt, bingeing, guilt, smoldering rage and emergency room visits. As a patient at the day treatment center she experienced counselors developing rapport and intimacy with her only to 'abandon' her with, what seemed in reviewing the case, alarming frequency. As a daughter to Margaret she was continually shopping for and attempting to please someone who seemed impossible to please.

We can see dissociation in Jenny's seeking help from various disparate providers, never allowing one to know about or talk with the other. She had relationships with various doctors who would treat her multitude of somatic complaints (heart disease, osteoporosis, migraine, arthritis, excess calcium and excess weight) but of course they were working in isolation from each other. She even had a separate personality in psychiatric treatment at a different rehabilitation center where she was seen by two different music therapists, while various counselors and therapists saw Jenny at our center.

Jenny's past, her internal world and her artwork were all filled with dissociated pieces. Things were being kept apart deliberately. Carey even stated that she used confusion to control Jenny. All of this dissociation, misery and confusion is seen as typically symptomatic of adult survivors of childhood trauma. The theories of Briere (1992), Herman (1992) and Shengold (1989) provide some understanding of Jenny's development and her way of coping with difficulties.

Briere (1992) focuses on the major types of psychological disturbances found frequently in adolescents and adults who were abused in childhood. He suggests that the sexual abuse survivor may have intrusive thoughts and/or memories of victimization, making it difficult for them to concentrate for extended periods of time and making it nearly impossible to have a 'nondistressing mental life'. These intrusive thoughts center around themes of 'danger, humiliation, sex, guilt, and badness. Intrusive memories usually involve unexpected and unwanted recollection of specific abusive or traumatic events in seemingly unrelated contexts' (Briere 1992, p.21). We have seen how these intrusive thoughts and memories interfered with everything about Jenny's life: cognitive functioning (her early artwork had a very childlike quality), the ability to relate to others (often giving them sadistic roles in her life story) and the ability to respond to life's stresses with some amount of balance.

Cognitive theorists point out that people make assumptions about themselves, others, the environment and the future based on the things they learned as children. If the child learns predominantly negative things she will grow up to have predominantly negative assumptions about herself and the world she finds herself in. She will be the victim of her own cognitive distortions. 'Abuse survivors may, for example, overestimate the amount of danger or adversity in the world, and underestimate their own self-efficacy and self-worth' (Briere 1992, p.23). When a child is assaulted it is not just an assault on the physical body but on her perception of her value, her competence and her view that the world is a generous place, or at the very least, a neutral place to live.

Often the abusive parents will justify their behavior by blaming and criticizing the child, rationalizing the abuse. This increases the child's feeling of badness. Briere talks about 'dichotomous thinking', this dichotomy being based on the child's primitive understanding of what is happening and of the parents' justification and blame. Briere suggests that the child will go through a thought process something like the following: I am being hurt by somebody I trust. This is because either I am bad or my parent is (the abuse dichotomy). I have been taught by others that parents are always right. If they do hurt me, it must be because I am bad. It must be my fault that I am being hurt. I must deserve this. I am as bad as whatever is done to me. I am bad because I have been hurt. I have been hurt because I am bad.

It is easy to see how the child with this way of thinking will grow into an adult who will continue to think this way, silently criticizing and disparaging herself. Her internal monologues will create feelings of helplessness and inadequacy, leaving her vulnerable to revictimization, which in turn confirms the learned helplessness and inadequacy, as we have seen repeatedly in Jenny's journal writing.

Herman (1992) addresses the idea that repeated trauma in adult life erodes the formed personality, but that repeated trauma in childhood necessarily 'deforms' the personality. The child trapped in an abusive, dependent relationship is faced with the task of adapting to this situation.

> She must preserve a sense of trust in people who are untrustworthy, safety in a situation that is unsafe ... Unable to care for or protect herself, she must compensate for the failures of adult care and protection with the only means at her disposal, an immature system of psychological defenses. (Herman 1992, p.96)

Herman describes the major forms of adaptation as being the elaboration of dissociative defenses and the development of a fragmented identity. These forms of adaptation permit the child to survive and to preserve the appearance of normality. The child can hide her distress within memory lapses and other dissociative symptoms, which often go unrecognized as the symptoms of abuse that they are. She talks about the child's formation of a malignant negative identity as being generally disguised by the socially conforming 'false self', which would perfectly describe Carey and Joy, Carey being harsh, punitive and destructive while Joy is a delightful, engaging, sweet identity.

Shengold (1989), in his discussion of abuse, talks about the representational world of the patient. He believes the space where patients interact with their therapists is their 'representational world', made up of mental images of the world inside and of the world outside the self. He believes victims find it very difficult to feel responsible for this representational world, their mental pictures of themselves or others, or the world around them. A child can register in her mind the experiences of having been seduced and beaten as well as fantasies of being seduced and beaten. She will believe that these mental pictures happen, not that she has created them. The parents, who are the first objects of the child's instinctual drives, do things to her and evoke things in her. All of this is registered within the child's mind and becomes a part of her representational world.

Shengold (1989), giving credit to drive theory, feels children are easily seduced because they want to be seduced. This is another reason for the child's belief that she is to blame for any mistreatment that befalls her, aside from Briere's discussion of dichotomous thinking. Children, after all, have an imperative need for parental attention and they will turn to seduction and provocation in order to get this attention. Their representational world will then be a confusion of memories and fantasies of seduction and abuse, resulting in their questioning their own stories and their own reliability.

Shengold then explains how the inflicting of trauma can seem to be passed down from generation to generation: 'For the developing infant, these gods of the nursery ... are the environment. They have power over the helpless ... They are also under a powerful unconscious compulsion to repeat the circumstances of their own childhood' (Shengold 1989, p.4). Shengold uses the concept of identification with the aggressor to explain this phenomenon, a way for the abuse survivor to 'be' the aggressor, to act out the memories and fantasies that are within her representational world. Jenny, for example, will not see the victim as a separate individual, she will not empathize with her victim, probably in the same way her mother was not able to see her as separate or to empathize with her. This identification with the aggressor will continue because of a 'need for rescue from unbearable intensities and defense against them' as well as a 'need to take on the attributes of the tormentor and turn on other victims the abuse that was suffered' (Shengold 1989, p.7). Identification with the aggressor is also a way of playing out the delusive wish to make the bad parent good. We see the child's resulting contradictory splits, fragmentation of impulse and identity, a confusion between victim and tormentor, between good and bad. We see the walled-off representations and mental compartmentalization: 'The child is motivated with compulsive force to avoid bringing the contradictory pictures together, the rage associated with the bad, which can overwhelm and destroy, must be kept away from the needed mental image of the good parent, but the rage remains' (Shengold 1989, p.30). The child's unconscious becomes a repository of murderous fantasy and impulse aimed at the parent and herself, compartmentalized and disconnected from consciousness.

Shengold sees our identity as a multidimensional web (a kind of Indra's net), consisting of introjected images from early childhood of parents and/or other important caretakers. These can be modified by succeeding important people in our lives. Shengold postulates that once past infancy we have an intense need for psychic synthesis, continuity and causality; a need to make sense of our internal and external world. 'What goes on within and without our minds may be ultimately unknowable; yet sanity and survival depend on comparatively accurate registration of the outer and inner worlds' (Shengold 1989, p.32).

Prior (1996) talks about a lack of theory for the understanding and treatment of the abused child, no shared assumptions, practices or inter-pretive ideas. He found most writing on the subject of abuse to be description of symptoms. In order to explain for himself why and how trauma and abuse distorts the dynamics and structure of the child's psyche, he turned to object relations theory. Although I don't agree that abuse and trauma literature are predominantly catalogues of symptoms, I do certainly agree that object relations theory brings one closer to a better understanding of how the human psyche, with all its representations, develops and is affected by relations with others and the environment.

Object relations

How do we actually develop these inner representations? Before I attempt to answer that question, I'd like to explain why I feel compelled to ask it.

Jenny's case material was shown to a family therapist who adheres to systems theory. After she read the case material she explained to me how easily the treatment could be explained in terms of systems theory, that Jenny was a product of several interrelated dysfunctional systems that needed to be deconstructed. Reparation occurs with the reconstruction of a more functional system, which happened to some degree in Jenny's treatment.

Robert Landy (1983 and 1986), the director of New York University's Drama Therapy Program, read the material and saw the obvious reparative value of Jenny's work on integrating various disparate roles. He said she had taken very rigidly held roles and revised or reconstructed them, exchanging various qualities, allowing for growth and change. He also acknowledged the power of puppets, dolls, objects, masks and make-up to foster healing through the creative use of imagination and projection.

As an art therapist I was interested in the reparative qualities in the art-making process, from Jenny's first depiction of her inner world to her final sculpture of Stewart (Figure 3.1), the music therapist. When I first asked if I could run a puppetry group at the center, my thinking was a puppet-making group. It seemed crucial that our patients be offered the opportunity to create their internalized object worlds in a more permanent, three-dimensional form, such as puppets. My assumptions were that this kind of art making provided an opportunity as well as a safe place where sublimation of un-acceptable impulses and drives could occur. As Edith Kramer (1996) said in reference to an adult survivor's use of art, 'Drawing pictures constituted a sanctuary of self-communication where the unthinkable and unspeakable could be given form' (p.72).

It would seem that this case material can be read and interpreted by clinicians of differing schools of thought. Each may see Jenny's growth in a slightly different way, perhaps attributing her improvement to different

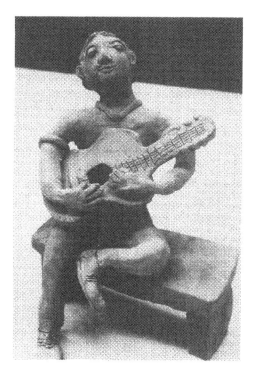

Figure 3.1 Stewart

aspects of her treatment; I suspect each may be correct in his or her vision, but I also suspect that each vision would not comprise the whole truth, only focus on an aspect of Jenny's treatment.

As a primarily psychoanalytically based art therapist I was curious about human development as seen specifically in creativity and body image development. What is beneath these positive effects of treatment? What does role theory have in common with sublimation and reconstruction? I believe each is an aspect of the creative process of Jenny's reparative movement in treatment. I believe her reparative urge informed everything creative that she did. I would like to understand this process better, this reparation that appears to alleviate the symptoms Jenny and others in her situation present.

I believe that how we develop as humans greatly depends on how our representational world develops; how we see things, how we interact with what we think we are seeing, how we hold the image of someone in our minds and how our childhood traumas still affect us today. I don't see this as a conflicting view with that of the systems theorists. I don't see this as conflicting with the drama therapist's role theory or with the art therapist's theory of sublimation. Object relations theorists write about how we develop our representational worlds and form symbols, how internalized objects are at the root of our various roles and how it is possible to repair or create a system that will serve or comfort us.

Object relations theorists construct their theories around the newborn infant and her relationship to the world. They begin with the idea of the maternal holding environment where the infant can feel perfect safety. The infant's needs are met, she is secure, warm and well fed. We can assume there was a time when Jenny experienced something similar. This experience of self and other is primarily a bodily experience. Ogden (1986) says, 'The newborn infant's world at the outset is a bodily world, and phantasy represents the infant's attempt to transform somatic events into a mental form' (p.11).

For normal development to occur, this holding environment needs to break down, to be imperfect, allowing the infant to enter what is called the paranoid-schizoid position. This normal and necessary disruption in the infant's perfect refuge where all needs are met, creates fearfulness. There are times when the infant might not feel perfectly safe, warm or well fed. She might develop a fear that the holding environment will not continue to go on being, a fear of annihilation of the mother upon whom she is completely dependent and a resulting fear of her own annihilation.

The way the infant manages this fearfulness is through primitive defenses, by splitting and isolating the loving and hurtful aspects of experience. It would be too dangerous for the infant to hate the object she loves, or love the object she hates, because she is completely dependent upon that object. She can't afford to lose it. Again, Ogden (1986) says, 'Splitting allows the infant … to love safely and hate safely, by establishing discontinuity between loved and feared aspects of the self and object. Without such discontinuity, the infant could not feed safely and would die' (p.64). Splitting creates safety by separation of the endangered from the endangering. It is also a way of ordering experience: good, bad, love, hate, me and not me. It is in splitting that we can assume the infant first begins to create some kind of internal image or mental construct in order to separate and order these aspects of self and other.

Projection can be seen as a form of splitting. The infant sees internal danger as different from internal soothing or comfort. She removes her internal danger and places it outside of herself.

Ogden believes that introjection can also be interpreted as a form of splitting. The infant sees the external object as split into endangering object and valued object. She places one or the other inside herself in order to protect the valued object. Denial, too, is a form of splitting, as when the infant treats a dangerous object as if it had been annihilated.

Projective identification is also a form of splitting, but in as much as it includes another person, it is an interpersonal elaboration of splitting. The infant projects her feelings onto the mother who, through her ability to contain these feelings, transforms them into meaningful experience, which is then reinternalized by the child. An example might be seen when a sympathetic mother talks to her crying, frightened or confused infant, explaining to her that she is hungry or wet, and miraculously the infant calms down. According to Ogden, as this defense continues to be used into adulthood, the individual may project split off, rejected aspects of the self in an attempt to 'take control' of another person from within. When observed in a therapeutic setting, what actually happens is the patient will put pressure on another to conform to her fantasy. We can see this more clearly in the hyper-vigilant adult survivor who needs to 'control' the other, the perceived potential abuser. When observed in a therapeutic setting, what actually happens is the patient puts pressure on another to conform to her fantasy. In Jenny's case we saw her repeatedly attempting to anger her counselors in order to get them to conform to her fantasy that they hated her and would abandon her. In as much as the therapist was able successfully to manage the feeling engendered by the patient, the patient would then have access to modified and manageable feelings. When I was able to say 'yes, this or that can make me annoyed, but that doesn't mean I'm going to quit my job and leave you', Jenny was able to understand that anger doesn't have to mean annihilation, that it can be manageable. Of course, the fact that her counselors did indeed keep leaving, presented obstacles in Jenny's ability to have access to modified and manageable feelings.

Developmental problems occur when the infant is unable to diminish her reliance on the defense of splitting as she physically matures. The result is a compartmentalization of life, of experience and of the self. Deri (1984) puts it clearly:

> ...without ... integrative symbolization, the environment is perceived as populated, on the one hand, by malevolent witchlike creatures and, on the other, by people of unreal perfection. The same person may also be perceived as two different entities, alternating between these two extremes. This is the split world of the borderline patient. (p.58)

Deri believes that if uncorrected by psychotherapy, the process of missymbolization deteriorates, leading to more and more threatening internal symbols until the world is seen as so threatening that aggressive acts of 'self-defense' are necessary.

She feels that the individual who lives in such a split world cannot be fully present in any given situation or relationship. There is always a sense of part of the self being missing, or behind a wall someplace. If, however, the infant has been able to split 'enough', to have enough of both positive and negative feelings and experiences without fear of annihilation, the groundwork is laid for eventual integration of part objects and parts of self. This didn't happen in Jenny's infancy or childhood. Jenny's environment provided constant threats of abandonment and abuse, often enacted on, so that her negative experience seemed to far outweigh any positive experience in both intensity and frequency.

If there had been relative freedom from the anxiety that loving experience will be contaminated or destroyed by hating experience, Jenny might have been able to bring these different facets of experience into closer relation with each other. The good object would no longer need to be kept quite so emotionally separate from the bad object. In Jenny's creation of puppets and dolls we did see the loosening of this rigidity in separation as the work recreated this normal developmental process.

With the integration of part objects and parts of self, with the lessening of the defensive use of splitting, we find the birth of the historical subject. This is considered by Klein to be the depressive position, but could easily be thought of as mourning. This is not quite as linear or rigid a process as Klein might suggest since we can observe children and adults moving between mourning and the fear and denial of her 'paranoid-schizoid position'. As the need to keep good and bad aspects of the self and others separate is lessened, gradually these things are understood to be good and bad aspects of the same thing. The black and white, good and bad, no-shades-of-gray quality of life found in the earlier state is exchanged for a full-toned, complex, multidimensional understanding of the self, the other, and the environment.

The child who has given up the black and white qualities of the schizoid position can become the interpreting subject 'I'. She can project her state of mind into her sense of the other and observe herself doing it. It is in this way that she begins to consider the possibility that other people experience feelings and thoughts in much the same way that she does, but that they are separate people. She can develop concern for others and is now capable of guilt and the wish to make reparation. Initially there was no guilt in Carey, only an impersonal ruthlessness and aggression towards Jenny and Joy.

In the later stage where mourning is possible one achieves whole object relatedness. The individual develops a sense of concern for people that they cannot control. They open themselves up for the possibility of being left by another person. There is a feeling of loneliness generated and maintained in this stage. The individual needs to tolerate this feeling without filling the void with projections of the self (as we see in the DID patient's creation of various alters) or in the creation of a paranoid world in which persecutory objects provide constant company.

Klein's depressive position is really about mourning the loss of object ties to that perfect maternal holding environment. Shengold (1989) says that humans live by metaphor, that they create poetry, myth and history. Once we leave infancy, we begin to 'weave our memories into narrative, from which we construct our identities' (p. 32), but we have to be willing to mourn the loss of infancy in order to leave it and we have to have had a balance of positive and negative experiences while in Klein's 'paranoid-schizoid' position, in order to move into the stage where mourning is possible. Mahler (1968) suggests that object constancy begins once the child is able to mourn the loss and begin to see people as whole and separate. Bergman (1996), however, reminds us that reaching the 'depressive position', like achieving object constancy, is a lifelong task and is not quite as linear as it may seem in writing and theory.

In Jenny's case we could observe her wish to maintain the inner drama and separation of Carey, Joy and Jenny. Akhtar, Kramer and Parens (1996) have suggested that resistance to change is a way to maintain stability. We observed Jenny's intense resistance to giving up the constant company of persecutory objects of her paranoid world. I saw my task with Jenny as to provide the balance needed between positive and negative experience, so that she would have the possibility to move from the 'safety' of that world of passivity and helplessness, into the sorrow and loneliness of the depressive position where she could begin to weave her memories into a narrative and to construct an integrated identity.

In order to help Jenny move away from her fragmented, part object world into whole object relationships I needed a clearer understanding of her inner representations of her self, her body image and of others. I suspected that the confusion of the race of her first two important 'other' puppets had something to do with her possibly not seeing the actual people as whole objects separate from her; Lisa, being an African-American puppet representing Dr Lisa, a white, Jewish psychiatrist, and Eric, an African-American puppet representing a blonde psychiatrist of Scandinavian descent. By the time she created the Lita puppet, painting an appropriate skin color to represent the counselor she was working with at the time, Jenny was beginning to differentiate, perhaps tentatively exploring the depressive position and seeing others as whole people with the range of color and nuance that it entailed.

Body image

Krueger (1989) addresses the issue of body self in human development. He suggests that although Freud recognized that ego development begins with the body ego, further study of the body and its evolving representation has been largely omitted from developmental and psychoanalytic theory. His interest came from working with patients with eating disorders, as well as other more severe narcissistic and borderline individuals. He observes that they lacked a consistent and accurate internal image of their bodies and sense of self. These patients would rely on other people and external feedback to create for them a sense of worth or adequacy. There was no object constancy and no self constancy. He also observed these patients using 'body self stimulation' to regulate affect, using food, drugs, alcohol, sex, wrist cutting, exercise and impulsive as well as compulsive behaviors. Being curious about the relationship between body image and development, he used serial projective drawings to elicit from these patients developmental data and reconstruction of their inner representations.

The central thesis arising from Krueger's work is that an individual's healthy sense of self contains, at its core, a cohesive, distinct and accurate body self. But if the individual's development is compromised it may be evidenced in an incomplete or distorted body self and image. He quotes Fenichel (1945): 'The sum of the mental representation of the body and its organs, the so-called body-image, constitutes the idea of "I" and is of basic importance for the further formation of the ego... (Krueger 1989, pp.3–4). Krueger speculates that the infant's body, feelings and movement are initially experienced through the mirroring of the mother. These experiences are assumed to coalesce into a body self awareness and then into a body image. He feels the development of an intact body image and the subsequent development of ego boundaries can be seen as occurring on a continuum: 'The baby is held, wrapped, touched, and supported. The boundaries thus defined have many qualities essential to the developing sense of self ... if there is overstimulation or understimulation, body self distortions ... begin, and may later result in narcissistic disturbances' (p.6).

He feels the internalization of the representation of the mother develops from these same consistent experiences. Krueger differentiates between the forming of the image of mother, which is produced in the psychic system, and perceiving the mother, which is derived from external visual stimuli. He postulates the infant's first symbol and the first transitional objects are those representing the body of the mother. He believes the very first transitional object is food, passed from mother to infant. The representation can be internally evoked without the mother's presence when the experiences are consistent, contributing to more constant, durable representations.

He characterizes normal body image development as being seen in progressively more complete, integrated body schema from infancy onward: 'The body image is a complex evolving formulation of an evocative mental representation of the body. Its developmental maturity is based on an individual's formation and perceptions of a series of internal and external stimuli' (Krueger 1989, p.11). Disturbances in the emergence of body self and psychological self, as we saw in the case material, occur when the sense of self-cohesion is threatened or has failed to develop. Jenny's preoccupation with bodily experience can be seen as a product of fragmented body self and psychological self, but also as 'an attempt to establish or restore a body integrity and representation' (Krueger 1989, p.40). Krueger theorizes that focusing on the body fulfills an organizing function for a fragmented ego, since the first and most basic organizer of ego experience is the body ego.

What comes to mind here is that not only did Jenny attempt to organize herself through her somatic preoccupation, but there were many art therapy sessions where she would place the little papier-mâché body parts in front of her and spend the entire session organizing and arranging them, with noted satisfaction. Jenny's somatic concerns actually seemed to me to be an expression of her introjected mother's 'bad', cruel and destructive qualities, thus populating her internal world with split-off persecutory objects. Watching Jenny arranging the papier mâché and cloth, creating little body image representations, however, seemed to have a more creative, generative, reparative quality. Krueger (1989) addresses the issue:

> ...the creative and expressive arts therapies offer more direct access to the unconscious and symbolic processes as well as to more basic experiences of the body self. The methodologies of expressive therapies allow direct experience of body self and basic affect without guilt by bypassing later developmental structures, such as superego, to directly access experience. (p.162)

Margulies (1989) also discusses body image and creativity. He feels the most primordial experience of self lives within the body ego, that 'the ineffable experience of the physical condensation of feeling, memory, pleasure, desire, ideals, anxiety ... all in a single and peculiar body-self sensation' (p.39). What he seems most interested in though is the evolution of self-change, of the opportunities for the self to conceive of the self anew: in other words, the therapeutic application of creativity to the image of the self, the opening of new possibilities of self-perception' (p.10). Is this what Jenny was doing with her body image representations?

From Margaret S. Mahler's (1968) careful observations of human development we can see body image development in terms of body-as-self developing gradually out of an undifferentiated phase in which feelings of being merged with the mother, 'a dual unity with one common boundary' (p.8), give way to differentiation. There is a growing awareness of boundaries and a growing ability to differentiate between inside and outside, between 'me' and 'not me', and one could assume a growing ability to take responsibility for one's thoughts and feelings (see the discussion of Shengold's work, above). All of the infant's growing skills (mouthing objects, pushing, grasping, kicking) can be seen in terms of their contribution to body image development. Of course, this skill learning doesn't take place in a vacuum. The infant has to mouth, push, grasp and kick something. The infant needs the maternal holding environment in order to develop the body-as-self.

Winnicott (1986) is well known for his discussions of the potential space and the maternal holding environment. He believed that much of the infant care, the holding, bathing, feeding and handling, serve to facilitate the baby's psyche-soma that lives and works in harmony with itself. He located healthy cultural experience in the potential space between a child and her mother when experience has shown the child that the mother can be counted on, that she will be there if needed.

If the child feels she can't count on the mother, as in Jenny's case where her mother left her in the hospital and then again on the court steps, there will be a disruption in the potential space, while traumatic experience will disrupt the harmony and integration of psyche and soma. The child requires an environment perceived as indestructible, but if the mother threatens abandonment, as in this case, the environment is perceived as uncertain and not to be trusted.

Winnicott (1986) observed, 'Opportunity for creative activity, for imaginative playing, and for constructive working – this is just what we try to give equally for everyone' (p.87). Perhaps the task of the art therapist is to create a potential space, an indestructible holding environment in the art room where the patient can work safely, creatively, imaginatively and constructively.

Susan Deri (1978), in an essay on the work of Winnicott, described a child's need to play in the presence of the mother. She says that in order for the child to play with enjoyment, the mother's main task is to create a play space, or transitional space in which her child can play and be alone in her presence. In this potential space – this good, creativity-fostering intermediate region, which both joins and separates mother and the playing child – the child feels 'unpressured by instinctual needs and unchallenged by the demands of the environment' (p.55). The mother can leave usable objects around without forcing them on the child. He will find and use what he needs. 'Finding them will be as much a creative act as the discovery of *objets trouvés* for the artist, or driftwood for the beachcomber' (p.56). The mother also watches the child play, her eyes and face function as a warm, friendly mirror, 'reflecting the loved image of the child to the child' (pp.56–57).

In describing the creation of a good-enough play space, Deri describes art room experience. The art therapist is always there, attentive enough to know what variety of tools might be useful so that the patient can find just the tool he or she might need. Watching seems very important, the confirmation that 'Yes, I know, art making is great.' This can be a look or a smile, nothing necessarily said. The work that is done reflects back to the patients that what they were doing was good, that who they were was good.

Giovacchini (1986) speaks of the analyst's need to survive the patient's destructiveness long enough for the patient to be able to perceive the relationship in terms of a holding environment that can survive her destructive fantasies and impulses. 'During treatment, a concretely oriented, unimaginative, and constricted patient may develop the ability to function creatively as he gets in touch with parts of the psyche that were previously in states of fragmented isolation' (p.12).

Like Margulies (1989), Giovacchini seems to be interested in how the patient is able to change. He speculates that the patient creates a new reality in the now benign holding environment, the transitional space, and incorporates it into her inner space, so that she can now gain control over what was previously seen as unpredictable and threatening. He sees the patient's remolding of reality and acquiring of new adaptations and controls as a creative achievement.

Finally, Clegg (1984) postulates the child's use of imagination in the recovery from developmental trauma particularly as it relates to transitional objects. In his analysis ideas, words, dreams and play may be interpreted as transitional phenomena vital to the healing process in general medicine as well as in various forms of therapy, such as art therapy. Therapists themselves can even be considered transitional objects since they foster communication between one part of the mind and another part. As he states: 'I will advance the hypothesis that transitional object phenomena are used in both the repair and the maintenance of healthy personality operations, that transitional objects are important in normal development and are particularly important in a child's therapeutic recovery' (p.33). It would seem that Jenny's art productions, particularly the body image representations, could be seen as transitional objects.

Clegg is particularly interested in reparation. He describes the classical Kleinian idea of reparation as the making amends to aspects of the other that the individual feels she might have damaged through her aggression. To that idea he adds the restorative actions to those aspects of the self felt to have been damaged by the patient's own greed, hate and aggression. As an example of this concept one can recall Carey periodically trying to make amends with Joy and Jenny. Clegg says, 'Reparation can thus be seen as involving the synthesis or linking of formerly split objects or, by extension, of formerly split object domains within the personality' (p.38). He cites Balint (1963) and Bloch (1978) as pointing out the necessity for good internal objects, that they are needed to combat the influence of inner threats as well as realistic external threats. In conclusion, Clegg states that our job as therapists is to recruit internal allies in the fight against persecutory fantasies.

I would like to end this discussion of theory with a quote from philosopher, magician and writer, David Abram (1996).

> If this body is my very presence in the world, if it is the body that alone enables me to enter into relations with other presences, if without these eyes, this voice, or these hands I would be unable to see, to taste, and to touch things, or to be touched by them – if without this body ... there would be no possibility of experience – then the body itself is the true subject of experience. (p.45)

Examination of treatment

If we go back to Jenny's story, using the theory just reviewed to examine her history and our work together, I believe we will gain a clearer idea of how she used art therapy. Starting with the maternal holding environment, we can assume that Jenny, as an infant, experienced a certain level of security and merging with Margaret, her mother. For the sake of this discussion we will assume that she had enough to eat and was held and bathed with enough care to result in the development of a body ego. We can also assume that things would take Margaret away from Jenny periodically. During these times she may have been perceived as the bad mother. We can hypothesize Jenny's rudimentary images and terror that the good mother might never return, that the source of all comfort and nurture was perhaps annihilated by something, perhaps the bad mother or even her own rage at the bad mother. However, Margaret would return and with her the holding environment, the transitional space in which Jenny could theoretically explore boundaries and develop her representational world in comfort and security. This comfort and security are critical for exploring and learning, while a lack of it creates annihilation anxiety, making it extremely difficult to take in information.

We now know that the holding environment needs to provide enough security for the infant to develop an internal source of comfort before it begins to break down, but we also know it needs to break down in order for the infant to develop beyond this symbiotic blissful state. I suspect that the holding environment that Margaret provided may have failed a bit too early and a bit too often for Jenny actually to form enough of a positive representational world for her personality to develop smoothly. From Jenny's description of her childhood, it sounded as though all of the important figures in her life – mother, father, older siblings – had a remarkable inability to empathize with her as a whole and separate individual, that they were all under their own pressures to identify with the aggressor. So we can assume that Jenny was having difficulty creating an internal source of comfort and that she was probably utilizing the early defense mechanisms of splitting, projection, introjection, denial, dissociation and projective identification. She would have been utilizing these defenses from her early childhood into her adult life when I began working with her. That constitutes quite a few years of practice, and one can see why these defenses were so well ingrained. One can also imagine the difficulty involved in moving beyond them.

Because of these defenses, her reporting and thus our understanding of her young adult years seems rather incomplete. Between the ages of 18 and 40 it seems that she completed a bachelor's degree in psychology or sociology (depending on who was telling the story), worked for the telephone company, got fired, worked for a church day care center, got fired and was brought up on charges of arson, would steal 'stupid things' like sheets once a month and not know why (according to her) and then began a series of hospitalizations and outpatient treatment at which point she came to the center where I was working.

In some ways the center continued to support her splitting, by providing her with a wide variety of treatment modalities, counselors and therapists. The center also continued to provide her with fuel for her abandonment panic, or annihilation anxiety, being a training facility where students and beginning therapists became accomplished and confident and moved on. We saw Jenny repeatedly lose her counselor, just when it seemed she had established a trusting relationship. The more this anxiety was fueled the more Jenny used her defenses. We could clearly see Jenny using splitting and dissociation between the art room and the pottery room. It was as if she were two completely different people in these two rooms. In the art groups and in puppetry she would often be a sulking, withdrawn, childish individual, while in pottery we saw an extremely competent, relatively outgoing and helpful individual.

Jenny was not the only patient to embody this change in personality. Many of the more antisocial borderline patients, as well as the patients suffering from narcissistic personality disorder, would go through a positive metamorphosis in the pottery room. I am sure the soothing tactile experience played a large part in this transformation. It is in the working with clay in this space that we can assume Jenny and others begin to experience something tactile, creative and positive. Even when an aggressive urge came into play, as when we saw Jenny fill a breast-shaped piece of clay full of holes, it could be turned into something useful, in this case a pencil holder, so that even one's destructive urges could somehow be absorbed by the clay.

One of the borderline patients had actually brought in an article from The New York Times about the ability of clay to absorb toxins and it was passed around among the group members with enthusiasm and interest. This clay did the same thing physically that it did psychologically. As Jenny projected her feelings into the clay, the clay was able to contain them, much as a 'good-enough mother' might, and then she was able to take them back, now in a less lethal form. This seems like a form of projective identification, especially when the art therapist is nearby and can point out how nice it is that the clay can take what looks like quite a bit of punishment and a lot of our negative feelings.

We could see this projection of internalizations in the art room as well. Jenny created many horrific pictures of her various internalized negative introjects, but primarily she created puppets and dolls to contain her projections. In fact, she could use the entire puppetry group in a kind of projective identification drama. When Mr Mad would express a desire for really hot chilies because he was such an angry puppet, the other patients in the group applauded. They mirrored Jenny's feelings, showed her that they were acceptable and that the group would not be annihilated by them. When Jenny threatened to put her counselor puppet in the 'City Dump: Home for Bad Puppets', the patients cheered, and even set up schedules when they would go and visit her in the Dump. The City Dump was actually a box created to contain the patients' transient negative feelings about a puppet, so that the patient could throw away a puppet but still know it wasn't destroyed. Before this box was created, the patients had been known to throw a puppet in the trash in a symbolic gesture that could result in its permanent damage from discarded paint, pencil shavings and coffee. The 'City Dump: Home for

Bad Puppets' was a good working solution. Many puppets came and went from that box, no worse for the experience.

Just as we saw that the art and pottery rooms provided a place for Jenny to project her feelings and then to reintegrate them, we saw that these two rooms provided her with a positive holding environment, a place where, when she was caught up in her abandonment and annihilation terror, she came and she knew these rooms would continue to go on being. At one point I asked her if she wanted to learn to use the kiln, a further effort to help her see her own competence and strength. She was very enthusiastic, admitting she was a fast learner. The kiln was at the very core of the magic of the pottery room. A piece would go into the kiln in a fragile, tentative state and then come out in a transformed solid state. Sometimes, though, as in life, things didn't always go well; the kiln would break down and become the 'bad mother', or more often a patient would have an air bubble in their piece creating terrible acts of destruction within the kiln which would be concrete expressions of the patients' destructive urges. The kiln would take this abuse and keep firing, so that the positive results always outnumbered the negative. On my vacations or absences from the center, being a part of the process of loading and firing the kiln was a great comfort to Jenny as it seemed for her possibly to support object constancy.

The art room and the pottery room provided Jenny with repeated opportunities to work on repairing or perhaps creating for the first time a whole body image representation as well as whole object relationships. The creation of artwork, puppets and dolls provided the physical mirroring that was so critical in the relationship between the infant and the mother. We could see her drawings develop from heads floating in space to full body drawings. We also initially saw her work at creating hand puppets that were not whole body representations, especially Mr Mad who was even without arms, to creating full body representations in the form of dolls, some of which were even self-representations.

As discussed above, the pottery groups provided Jenny with the comforting physical activity of holding, patting, touching and supporting (all the ingredients involved in the infant's development of body ego). One patient said in Jenny's presence, 'clay is very forgiving, that you could cut off an arm and attach it many times and it would always forgive you, where as a person probably would not' (Gerity 1997, p.93).

Jenny could experiment with little papier-mâché body parts, attaching, pulling apart, reattaching and in the process experiment with the representation of self-cohesion, which was something that in her childhood was always under threat and because of her use of primitive defenses continued to be under threat. Through art Jenny could experiment with object constancy, much as we see infants pulling their little 'Velcro' dolls apart and then reassembling them.

We see that the art therapist was able to provide a consistent holding environment, the necessary potential space in which Jenny could play, imagine and hope. She insisted that I create the box that was home for the dolls that represented her various parts as children. She picked the colors for the outside and the cloth for the inside, but it was my job to put it all together. She even maneuvered the interviews with the dolls so that I was putting them away at the end of the session. Towards the end of this documented year she began to take responsibility for them and care for them, putting them away herself. She was also eventually able to create her own transitional objects in the form of the dolls' quilts like the ones that her great-grandmother had made.

In her clay work, we saw an expression of sheer physical joy in a sculpture of a mother salamander with its babies crawling all over it (Figure 3.2). Each little creature is absolutely radiant with bliss. Then we have the final expression of whole body image: the three-dimensional portrait of the music therapist with his guitar (see again Figure 3.1). This piece had gone through its own periods of destruction and ultimate reparation. We see a somewhat wistful expression on his face as if he knows how difficult it is to leave those you care about and how difficult it is to be left, and yet there is an acceptance in this expression. He holds his guitar, which might be seen as a disguised body image representation of Jenny with its feminine curves and sense of emptiness at the heart of it. I believe this piece, with its destruction and recreation, assured Jenny of her own ability to make reparation, to create an expression of her object constancy and to reveal her grief as well, with the assurance that neither she nor the object would fall apart.

In concluding this review of Jenny and her passionate attachment to art therapy, I believe that by examining the documented changes in Jenny's behavior as well as, in her artistic processes and products, evidence of changes in body image representation over time, we saw that some of the benefits and improvements in this case could be associated with the application of experiences in art therapy. However, given the complexity of the human mind, with its history, 'hard wiring' and conditioning, as well as the complexity of her treatment, with all of the various doctors, counselors

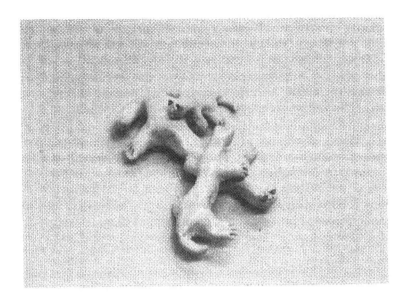

Figure 3.2 Salamanders

and therapists, it would be impossible to determine exactly how much of her improvement was due to her work in the art room and how much was due to other influences. Clear benefit, though, was observable within the context of art therapy.

Recalling that Jenny was initially unable to form a complete representation of self as a unit, I would suggest that some of her improvement was associated with use of art materials to explore the possibility of representing self as a unit within a safe and consistent environment. Her work in pottery seemed to provide the safe starting place, the holding environment that she could return to whenever she needed. It was here that through her slab work she first began to put various pieces together to make a whole, and this was practiced many, many times. The puppetry group provided a place to begin to externalize and work with the internal object world, and art groups gave her materials and the place to explore and integrate various parts of her body image, her sometimes frightening inner world and her external world.

An elegant example of this integrating process can be seen in a pencil drawing of an apartment building Jenny created to represent her internalized object world. She created this in response to a group member's questioning of how her various personalities fit together. Mr Mad and his family live at the very top of an apartment building. On the next floor down, Joy, Carey and Little Carey live. On the floor below we find Lisa and her baby, swinging his bottle out the window by his teeth. Below her are Eric and Lita, and at the ground floor we find Jenny guarding the front door. Scattered throughout the building are shuttered windows, as yet not revealing who lives behind them. On a separate piece of paper, split off from the building itself, is the basement (or the unconscious) where we find Jenny's mother, Margaret, with her spiky-haired guard, Sebastian. Margaret has what looks like an unusually large collection of goods and supplies: blankets, jars and bottles of food and drink, drawers and cabinets of hidden contents, as well as a refrigerator and freezer. Jenny was able to make some order of how these parts of herself all fit together in a more objective way than was possible in puppetry alone. Both puppetry and art worked together to reveal to Jenny what she was working to integrate, something that pottery could not have done alone.

I think by looking at this combination of Jenny's inner processes and the artistic products in depth and over a period of time, we can see reparative activity in various forms of art therapy. Simply asking Jenny what internal changes she perceived herself going through seemed simplistic and open to subjective bias. Interpreting her artwork alone, without her input, would also be simplistic and bias ridden. I needed a window into Jenny's world, a place where we could talk and exchange ideas in a non-threatening, non-invasive manner.

Intuitively, I reached for the puppets. This was a fortuitous act on my part, for not only was this now a place for us to talk about what the reparative qualities of art were for her, but it clearly became a therapeutic tool or technique in its own right, a playful, creative interchange where anything might happen.

We saw in interviews and in Jenny's journals that she was interacting with her inner representations. We saw how she took a transitional object, Sweet Basil, and turned her into a member of her internal object world. She then created little dolls to represent her child 'selves' and was able to treat them with the care she felt was lacking in her actual childhood. With all of this interaction and internalizing good objects, Jenny's characters became less fixed in their states. Because the characters were externalized into an art form, the puppets could grow and change, metaphorically representing the growth and change that was occurring internally as well.

One might worry that since a puppet may represent a dissociated part of the person, wouldn't such play encourage and concretize the different parts? I think this concern was underlying the music therapist's directive to 'get rid of Jenny'. However, the patient is the puppeteer, identifying with the role of the one in control. As a puppeteer she projects these parts into an art form and manipulates them, instead of using them as a defense and being manipulated by them. Most significantly, and in a spirit of play, Jenny was able to go beyond the parts in her identification with the puppeteer role, which can be seen as a metaphoric expression of the integrated self.

Can what was learned from Jenny be applied to the other 'adult survivor' patients who used art therapy? As Krueger (1989) discusses, a healthy sense of self contains a cohesive body self and individuals whose development was compromised by abuse and trauma contain a less than healthy cohesive body self. Some of these individuals were using the art room and materials found there to repair (or perhaps even generate in some cases) a cohesive, healthy body image representation and a stronger sense of self. Because of this close examination of work with Jenny, I was able to improve my treatment of others. I was better able to see and accentuate the indications of growth and change.

In working with imagery in the art room, these patients found a voice and a way to speak of things that were unspeakable. Through drawings and paintings their sense of self could look back at them from the paper. Art was a window into the inner world and through this window individuals gained a better understanding of who they were. In pottery, the shattered sense of self could be projected into the clay and put back together with 'slip' and care. In puppetry, the actual physical creation of puppets further strengthened the patients' body image formation through the same projective process. They could also bring more flexibility to their once rigidly held roles or dissociated personality-parts through playful and creative interaction. This flexibility was expressed in the continual renovation that the puppets underwent. I would venture to speculate that one of the most therapeutic qualities of puppetry, though, was that the patient was identified with the role of puppeteer and was therefore in charge of all the various puppets and the parts that they represented. The patient/puppeteer was enacting the workings of a healthy sense of self, one that has a repertoire of roles that can be used when needed, with grace and agility. Most importantly, however, is the fact that the patient as puppeteer is *conscious* of the roles that his or her puppets represent and consciously *chooses* when and how to employ them.

In the chapters that follow, I would like to introduce the various stories, characters and healing metaphors that emerged from the puppetry group. We have examined the therapeutic process within one case, but the things learned from this one case can be broadened out into a group setting. We have seen how body image is central to the healthy sense of self and the role this plays in the creation of puppets, but now I'd like to introduce the idea of metaphor and narrative and the weaving of story into art to augment the therapeutic work done with body image representation.

During the early 1990s, when our agency's funding was being reduced, the various therapists would try to assert the essential nature of the work they did and I was no exception. I would state that the traumas these patients suffered were more often than not preverbal and that the most effective therapeutic modalities would be ones which worked on those preverbal trauma memories. In retrospect, though, I see that the problems and symptoms are actually very complex and that the more avenues available to do therapeutic work the better. Puppetry, because it works on various levels with a variety of modalities at once, has the potential of being a very powerful therapeutic tool. In the following chapters we will see the power of story and narrative to help individuals begin to create a feeling of tribe, to begin to work together towards creating integration of self in community.

Shengold (1989) said that humans live by metaphor, that we create poetry, myth and history, that we begin to 'weave our memories into narrative, from which we construct our identities' (p.32). I would like to present other 'survivors' and their narratives, fictional narratives created around puppets, from which they were able to construct new possibilities and hope. I trust that it will become clear that these narratives were used in this reparative, generative way by the patients, both at an individual level and at a group level.

CHAPTER 4

Metaphor and Story

'Anything Can Happen in Puppetland'

The theory

> Throughout history, myths and metaphors have played an important part
> in education and in the development of wisdom. (Lankton and Lankton
> 1989, p.xv)

In the field of family therapy there is a growing interest in the use of narrative in therapy. White and Epston (1990) are well-known proponents of 'narrative therapy'. They base their work on the early work of anthropologist Victor Turner, who explored the ritual process of marking the different stages that humans go through at various points in their lives. These stages can be choreographed, ritualized rites of passage or simple stages a person goes through at a crisis point in their life. They include separation, liminality and reincorporation. Turner (1974) examined various cultures and found these stages to be a fairly universal way of giving meaning to life events. In their practice, White and Epston have developed rituals to create rites of passage as a part of the therapeutic process. They have incorporated Turner's stages as part of their treatment, suggesting that clients look at their lives as anthropologists and create narratives and meanings from what they find. White and Epston encourage their clients to put these life events onto a mythic plane where meanings can change, where narratives can be transformed and transforming, and where they can again find hope.

How does creating a narrative about suffering and loss help an individual? Is it the making of meaning that is in itself therapeutic? Or is it the stepping outside of one's personal suffering and seeing the context, seeing the world and one's place in it? There is an old Buddhist tale that is a wonderful example of the power and importance of narrative. This is a story of one woman's suffering and her finding of meaning in it.

> A woman's only son died and she was so grief stricken that she carried his body about with her, asking everyone she met for help to restore his life. Someone directed her to the Buddha, and she asked him to please restore her son's life to his body. The Buddha said with reluctance that yes, he could do that, but he would need a special seed, a mustard seed from a house that has known no suffering. The woman set off eagerly to find this seed. She went from house to house, looking for a house that had known no suffering. In each house she heard a story, a narrative of suffering. After traveling for a long, long time and talking with many, many people she returned to the Buddha and said that she realized that suffering and loss are a part of life, and that her son's death had been a kind of gift, opening her heart to the suffering of others. She was really able to see others, to hear their stories with compassion, that she now felt awake where she had once walked in a dream. And the sharing of the stories, the sharing of suffering had eased her pain. Her compassion for them had served as compassion for herself as well. (A version of this story can be found in Goldstein and Kornfield 1987, p.87.)

Being an art therapist, I came late to the idea of narrative and story as something used in the context of therapy. However, working with patients in puppetry gave me a sense of respect for the possibility that stories can strengthen the therapeutic work we do. The patients used their puppets to enact rites of passage, to create stories that represented their own lives, much as White and Epston and even Turner described. They were doing this and creating a sense of community, creating group myths and characters. Because of the art-making component, there was a very real object constancy about this community. Stone (1996) described a communal story experience from West Africa called 'Ladder to the Moon'. Villagers would gather around a central fire in the evening as the stars appeared in the night sky, and the stories told moved slowly from the events of the day to stories of the ancestors. 'Onward through the night the stories are woven together, legends giving way to folk tales, then to wonder tales filled with magic and mystery' (p.60). This describes the creation of a communal weaving of story, entailing careful listening and a kind of building on what was heard, until a 'Ladder to the Moon' is completed.

The narratives and journeys that emerged from the puppet-making group were a courageous attempt to move beyond blame and projections for their life situations. For most of these patients trauma had caused them to isolate themselves from others, and they sometimes seemed very much alone and alienated, even among people who obviously cared about them. They appeared to shut down more and more aspects of themselves, more and more avenues of exchange with the world. In puppet making, though, something changed. Like the story of the woman looking for a mustard seed from the home that had known no sorrow, they began to look around themselves, listening to the stories of others' puppets. They began to see that they were not alone at all, that through opening their awareness they entered a kind of mythic plane, or a Winnicottian transitional space, dubbed Puppetland. This group gave the patients an opportunity to look at their life's journey in a larger context, to create community, to build 'Ladders to the Moon', to feel awake where they had been in a dream.

Alexander

I will begin with Alexander's story and those that emerged around his puppets. I had often heard him say 'anything could happen in Puppetland', an optimistic statement about the world of imagination. One time, caught up in a didactic frenzy, he took a pencil and drew two large, overlapping circles on the brown paper that covered the tables. He shaded in the oval formed by the overlapping circles. 'OK,' he said once he was sure he had the group's attention, which he did, ' this circle is us.' And he wrote 'us' in one circle. 'And this circle is reality,' he said, as he wrote 'reality' in the second circle. 'And this bit,' pointing to the shaded oval, 'this is Puppetland.' And he wrote 'Puppetland' in large letters across the top of his two overlapping circles. 'This is where anything can happen.' He could have been giving a lecture on Winnicott's 'transitional space', explaining how the child's inner world is right there next to the good-enough mother and how the area of overlap, the area of cultural experience or play, is the place where 'things can happen'.

Alexander had not always sounded so hopeful, though. As an adult survivor of childhood trauma, he held on to his self-protective rage along with his role of victim for many, many years. He had been raised by, from his report, a seductive borderline personality disordered mother. There were fabrications and uncertainty surrounding his father and the subsequent boyfriends that his mother entertained. He had first come to our center in his late adolescence, an extremely angry young man. During the ten years that followed, he developed a reputation as the worst neo-Nazi, hateful, frightening borderline patient one could work with. Psychiatrists dreaded their appointments with him, he had been asked to leave every verbal group he had ever been a part of, he was one of the patients that Herman (1992) said evoked 'unusually intense reactions … Sometimes they are frankly hated' (p.123). He trusted no one, had little sense of object constancy, and struggled with alcoholism and agoraphobia. As a kind of last chance it was suggested that he try art therapy.

The prospect of Alexander coming to art groups was terrifying. Pushing down my fear, I showed him where the materials were kept and told him that whatever he did in the art room was okay as long as it was on the paper. Alexander seemed to appreciate having this place where self-expression was really allowed, even encouraged. He gradually became a regular in many of the art groups during the week and after many, many pictures of guillotines, bombings, death and destruction, he slowly allowed others within the art room to see a less hostile aspect of himself. Here he was able to work quietly and expressively, but each piece seemed self-contained, each session seemed isolated and removed from the reality of his life, as if the art room were a sanctuary that needed to be kept split off and protected from the danger of the 'real world'. He would talk about the real world 'impinging' on him and that the art room was his refuge. I began to notice on some days when the world had 'impinged' with a bit more ferocity, he wore an SS ring that signaled to people to stay away. This splitting of the real world and the sanctuary reminded me of a popular television show at the time, *Beauty and the Beast*. When the Beast was in his sanctuary underground he was a warm, generous Beast. When he was above ground in the real world of Manhattan, he was a fearsome Beast and his claws and teeth showed. I knew that Alexander watched this show religiously, so I observed the relationship between himself and the character, the Beast. I observed that when he wore the SS ring it was on days when he was feeling the world's encroachment on his life. By acknowledging the changes, the splitting of a good world and a sanctuary off from the real world of violence and aggression, I hoped to bring some of this splitting into consciousness. I hoped to begin to find a way to help him integrate these various split-off parts of the self.

When he asked if he could join puppet making, I was delighted, even relieved. I saw from my work with Jenny that this modality provided great potential for integration and a real way to anchor gains and growth.

Indeed, it seemed the things Alexander and the other group members learned in puppet making could be integrated into their lives. Myths, a sense of history and context, were woven around the puppets. Their stories grew or evolved from week to week and the creators would carry the stories beyond the confines of the art room, musing over the meaning while riding the subway or cooking a meal. Lankton and Lankton (1989) suggest that stories are things we recall and ponder. Alexander used images well, expressing much of what had been inexpressible, but now he was creating something else with the image, a narrative that could be reflected upon and linked to his 'real' life.

Through participating in this group Alexander experimented with various parts of himself and with new ways of interacting. He was able to create a narrative to explain his puppet Rigvan's reactions to the world, and by doing that his own suffering and motivations became clearer to him. He found it much easier to talk about Rigvan's fears and shame than his own, so he spoke for Rigvan with empathy, discovering that within his own imagination lay possibilities, generosity and caring. It gradually dawned on him that Rigvan's difficulties were very like his own and that he actually felt a great deal better when he found solutions for Rigvan.

Alexander helped to create a sense of community, and to define the space that was christened Puppetland, a kind of holding environment complete with imaginary, flexible boundaries which seemed to go beyond the art room or the limits of time, history and culture. As with Jenny and her puppets, it was through Alexander's puppet that we began to see beyond his frightening persona. We now had a way of communicating with him, a window or a doorway through which we could meet and talk. But perhaps I should let the puppets tell their own stories.

I will tell you the stories of Puppetland, as they were told to me. Puppetland was a mysterious place where human people and puppet people could meet and play together. We would sit around a fire, late into the night, listening to each other's tales. Now I will tell of Rigvan, Vedrina and their human friend Alexander.

Rigvan's story has elements of bitterness and of triumph. Staring into the fire, he spoke vaguely about a happy childhood in the Ukraine, but then came the shadow and cold of the Siberian work camps which were unspeakable in their horror. Speaking with difficulty, he described the pain of frostbite. Workers were forced to cut down trees in sub-zero weather in their pajamas. It was while cutting down those trees that he made a vow to himself that one day he would be free, that he would be warm and his stomach would be filled. As he talked about these things, he seemed to be in a trance. He told us of how a woman in the cell next to his was beaten, tortured and raped, of how he could do nothing to help her, of how he was forced to listen helplessly. And this woman was his mother. After saying that he fell silent for a long time. Rigvan truly knew the meaning of regret and sorrow.

But he had a hunter's fire in his heart. He overcame the ice and oppression of Siberia and came to America. Rigvan said he blessed that day. This he could speak of easily and often, how this was a land of great opportunity, freedom, goodness and safety. 'You can make a real killing on Wall Street,' he was fond of saying, having grown comfortable with the American idiom. The fire in his heart led him to acquire a sizable import–export business as well as an estate in an area where the boundaries of Long Island and Puppetland overlapped. These triumphs had not taken away the pain and regret from the memories of the work camps, however, so he tried to numb that pain and wall it off with the finest firewater available, to no avail. Fate, being a capricious thing, provided him with great suffering as well as the opportunities to learn and thrive, but he had to be awake to act on them.

One day he met Vedrina, one of fate's opportunities, and as soon as they saw one another they knew that there was a story to be created between them, a story of promise and future. It was a very momentous day for all of the puppets, in fact, the day of the Great Hunt.

It was called the day of the Great Hunt because Rigvan's friend Ungar urged them to go into the wilderness (on Rigvan's estate) with their bows and arrows. But I should explain who Ungar was, first. He was a warrior puppet who had gotten caught in an ice floe long ago. Separated from his tribe and frozen for many, many years, when a thaw finally came he found himself alive but without a tribe. What else could he do but come to Puppetland? Ungar met Rigvan and they immediately recognized the fire of the hunter in one another. Together, on Rigvan's estate, the two would mount horses and hunt in the forest with bow and arrow. Time passed and Rigvan taught Ungar the customs and the things that puppets hold most dear; freedom, friendship and the sharing of a good story and food over the campfire.

On one particular day a puppet called Victoria forgot about some of the customs of Puppetland. She found her heart full of poison. With poison in her heart there was no room for caring about freedom, friendship or sharing. She attacked Rigvan, knowing that if he defended his honor they might fight to the death. She was willing to risk this, even hoping it would come to pass to assuage this darkness in her heart. She was in the foulest of tempers. As it happened this was also the day that

Vedrina arrived in Puppetland, with her long black hair and blue fur cloak. Rigvan had come to a difficult place, being ready to fight for his honor to the death, and yet here was this new and most interesting puppet, Vedrina. What was he to do? Ungar, being a quick-thinking friend, suggested that Rigvan quietly let Victoria know that she had forgotten the customs of Puppetland rather than actually fight to the death with her, and that they could then take the fire of revenge that was flowing through their veins and go on a hunt, a great bison hunt. Rigvan sighed with relief at this perfect solution, agreed with Ungar immediately, and added that Vedrina should be their tracker. This would allow Rigvan the opportunity to learn more about this mysterious black-haired puppet. The hunters' passion was great, 47 bison were killed, and the tribe was well fed for many months. The balance of the tribe was maintained. All was well.

In the story of Rigvan, Alexander was able to describe the helplessness and misery of his adolescence. He placed Rigvan in a Siberian work camp where he was forced to suffer physically as well as emotionally, where he was paralyzed in his inability to help his mother. Rigvan's great excitement at finding freedom in America and on Wall Street paralleled Alexander's gratitude at finding the art room and, more specifically, the puppet-making group. The freedom of expression that he found in that group was, to him, priceless. At last this was a place where he could trust others, until the day Victoria's puppeteer came into the session looking for someone to fight. The group leaders actually came prepared. We had been warned that a fight was brewing between these two. I'd brought in the mysterious female puppet with black hair and blue fur cloak (Figure 4.1). Another therapist, Du Rand, decided that her puppet, Ungar, would take Rigvan on a hunt if he was willing, so that Alexander would be able to 'experience … contain and work with his rage with some awareness ' (Du Rand and Gerity 1996, p.10). The awareness could occur because he knew Rigvan was a representation of himself.

Both of the interventions worked very well; the hunt was a great success and Alexander seemed genuinely delighted to find this female puppet which he immediately named Vedrina and began speaking through. It seemed to give him an outlet for a softer voice, a kinder aspect of himself that was interesting to him, something new and unexplored. So Vedrina and all she represented became a reason to stay, a reason to maintain the balance of the group, to avoid a battle to the death, or the eviction from the group. The hunt

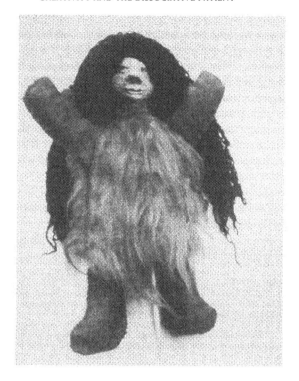

Figure 4.1 Vedrina

provided an outlet for the rage, a socially acceptable one. The tribe was well fed for months to come. Vedrina and Rigvan's story continues.

Vedrina and Rigvan had a sparkle in their eyes when they looked at one another or spoke about one another. When other puppets asked if they were married, Rigvan was fond of saying that their relationship was much deeper than that of marriage, that it was a business partnership. One spring, Vedrina looked about her and saw that some puppets were producing baby puppets. Her friend Alexander had made a comment to her about the size of her hips being good for childbearing, so, before anybody knew what happened, she and Rigvan had a little son, Nicholas. For many puppets it was a profitable and creative spring that year. Anything could happen in Puppetland.

Now after a time, although Rigvan was most happy with his family, he began to suffer blackouts from the firewater because he was still trying to numb the pain of the memories. He found that the firewater only took away the pain for a short time and when its effects wore off his pain was doubled. And there was Nicholas to think of. Rigvan was a good father and did not want to sleep through his son's childhood. So he consulted his travel agent and they decided he should take the waters in the finest spas in Europe where he could dry out in comfort. He could also entertain his mind with the history and culture of the lands through which he traveled. The last and best spa he visited was in Split, Yugoslavia, on the Adriatic Sea. This was a quest, and he marked his return with new clothes made by a little Ukrainian seamstress down on the Lower East Side.

We will hear more of Rigvan's and the rest of the tribe's stories in later chapters. How these stories effected change was a mysterious process for the group members. Sometimes they would put their puppets down and talk about the subversive qualities of the process, that they could feel things shift and change and that the myths which they shared were a way of passing on the things that they had learned. Bettelheim (1977) was interested in how fairy tales are understood by children and how they actually can help a child develop. We can see, though, that what is true for the development of children is true also for adults and that what Bettelheim writes about fairy tales is true also about the myths that emerged from this group.

> Each fairy tale is a magic mirror which reflects some aspects of our inner world, and of the steps required by our evolution from immaturity to maturity. For those who immerse themselves in what the fairy tale has to communicate, it becomes a deep, quiet pool which first seems to reflect only our own image; but behind it we soon discover the inner turmoils of our soul – its depth, and ways to gain peace within ourselves and with the world, which is the reward of our struggles. (Bettelheim 1977, p.309)

Lankton and Lankton (1989) were also interested in how myths and metaphors have been a part of the development of wisdom. The stories that emerged in this puppet-making group helped the puppeteers develop parts of themselves that were thought to be lost or sleeping. These tales of awakenings and things found were of their own creation and were accepted as pools of wisdom that they could learn from. Solutions to problems were found within these stories.

In this chapter, in Alexander's struggles, we have seen a development from immaturity to maturity. We have seen sublimation of the aggressive, self-destructive drive into a great hunt and feeding of the tribe. Rigvan went from being an isolated puppet, freezing, tortured and helpless in the Gulags, to a puppet capable of finding warmth and generosity of spirit in others and himself. Through the making of puppets and the creating of their stories Alexander found object constancy, a trust in the ongoing quality of life, that things learned in the group could be applied elsewhere, that things did not have to be walled up, split off, or protected quite as fiercely as they once did.

Once, during a particularly happy celebration, Rigvan turned to the Wise Old Woman's apprentice, who was called Artemis, and said he wished he could somehow bring Alexander to Puppetland permanently, that maybe Alexander could be happier then. Artemis reminded Rigvan that Alexander carried the images of his puppets within him and that this gave him comfort during hard times. Rigvan pondered this for a moment and then agreed.

CHAPTER 5

Transference and Splitting
The Abyss – Self and Community

In this chapter we will explore the abyss beneath Puppetland. The abyss was filled with the fears and projections of the adult survivor. These fears and projections were called transference and splitting by the staff; this gave us a sense of mastery over such things, or at least a false sense of security, believing that because we could name it in the patients we were free from its grasp.

In order to understand the process more clearly I will introduce Susan and Crystal, two women who had survived childhood trauma. If asked about these two women, most staff and clients would refer to their physical beauty. They were both very good at attractively making themselves up to subtly accentuate their fine features, both very focused on the surface appearance of things which the people around them then reinforced, although not intentionally. Crystal was a blonde with long, flowing hair that she could swish about dramatically and Susan was brunette with a perky, shoulder-length bob and long bangs from under which she would peek out coyly. They were able to capture the attention and focus of even the most self-involved psychotic patient. An interesting fact was that they could not be in the same group – they could not tolerate one another. But separately, each was a very lively group member, articulate and helpful. In verbal groups they would act as if they were there to assist the leader, always coming up with good insights, presenting themselves as model patients. 'I want to set a good example,' Crystal once said in a confidential tone. With enthusiasm the staff looked forward to having them in their groups, at least in the beginning. This is where we begin to see the dawning of transference and counter-transference.

The verbal groups seemed to be useless in helping Susan or Crystal gain mastery over their way of viewing the world. For them the world was clearly divided between those who had power and those who did not. If you were a group leader, you had the role of parent in the group and you had power. If you were a group member, you had the role of child and you had no power. Clearly it would be best, according to their world view, to be the group leader and have power.

After the initial honeymoon phase with Crystal and Susan, we began to ask why they were there. We would ask about their stories and what the group could give them. They might then pull out a fossilized rendition of an initial trauma, and possibly the fossils of further trauma. These stories had a very rigid feel to them, as if they had been pulled out before, to justify their feelings towards those who had wronged them, or to justify their beliefs in the world being the way they saw it. These stories had been formed long ago and would not have been so destructive if they were 'just' stories, but they had become the way that Crystal and Susan saw the world. They would interact with others based on their memories.

In these fossil memories, both Crystal and Susan were powerless, helpless, while the abuser was felt to be powerful. In the retelling they presented themselves as helpless while the group leader was seen as the powerful person in the group. We didn't have the tools in verbal groups to examine this process. We quickly became caught in the transference. Because we asked about the story and because the retelling had opened old wounds and recreated the old dynamic, the group leader was seen as the bad object, the perpetrator, or the aggressor. At this point the group leader would find themselves to be on the bad side of the split world view with no means of redemption. However, the language of Puppetland did provide the tools to explore these very difficult areas and it is the participation of Susan and Crystal in puppetry that we will now examine.

Susan worked very hard in puppetry. She recreated, through puppets, the various aspects of herself, or her internal object world. She had a helpless, ineffectual mother named Measle (Figure 5.1), a wailing, abused toddler (Figure 5.1), a competent but angry tomboy character (Figure 5.2), and the aggressor, who looked like a saber-toothed, red-faced devil (Figure 5.3). These puppets had little interaction with the other group members' puppets. Susan was very focused on the group leader for approval, as if no one else in the group existed. She engineered the use of the center's video equipment to create a film with her puppets outside of the group. This was at a time when

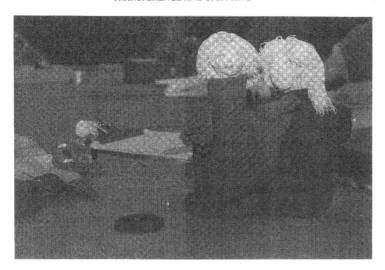

Figure 5.1 Measle and the toddler

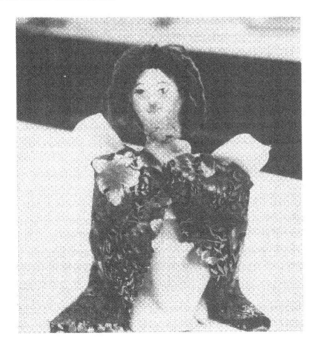

Figure 5.2 The angry tomboy

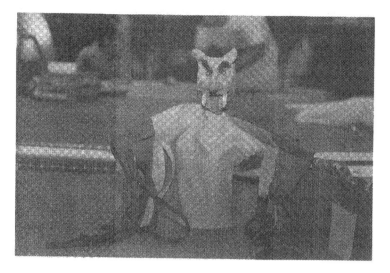

Figure 5.3 The abuser

we were being told that dissociative patients need to connect memories to feelings, so after some discussion between staff members, Susan was entrusted with the equipment. The resulting video was dynamic and expressive. She was pleased with herself and her obvious talents. She may have gained some mastery over the early trauma, connecting some affect to memory, but these things were not the entire reason for creating the video, in fact it was simply a means to an end. She was still seeking the approval of or merging with the group leader, the perceived source of power. When this did not happen she became very frustrated. I fell into the bad half of the split world view.

This was puppetry, however, and we had a metaphoric language to begin to understand these less than conscious processes. During one session we set up a drama in which Susan could direct the puppets. We used a wooden stage that had been created by one of the group members in a woodworking group. The group members played the role of the Greek Chorus, reminding us of what puppets can and can't do and what puppeteers can and can't do.

> The curtain rises on the toddler in the center of the stage, crying. We see the abuser, with his red face and saber-toothed grin, as he hovers and swoops over the toddler. The abuser can fly, streamers of red and yellow fluttering from his arms, as he laughs with a deep, frightening voice.

Then he flies off when he sees Miss Pie, a baker of pies, coming on stage. She sees the toddler and asks the child what is wrong (Figure 5.4). The child is not able to talk. All she can do is cry. Miss Pie wants to know if someone has hurt the toddler. She just cries and then Miss Pie wants to know if she'd like a nice big piece of fresh-baked pie with milk. (This is her solution to all of life's twists and turns.) At this point the tomboy enters the stage, full of bluster and judgement.

'What's wrong with you, a piece of pie, can't you see the toddler has been hurt? Disgusting little brat,' she mutters and then sharply demands, 'Who hurt you?'

(All of this is being watched with rapt attention by the group.)

Of course, the toddler says nothing. Then Measle is placed on the stage (resting on a cone so that she can be on stage without being manipulated by Susan) and the tomboy begins to berate her.

'What's the matter with you that you let your little kid get hurt,' the tomboy wants to know. Measle is terribly inarticulate, very similar to the toddler in fact. She whines and says she doesn't know how to take care of the toddler.

'Maybe someone else should take care of the toddler, maybe Miss Pie should,' Measle suggests, whimpering.

At this point the Greek Chorus pipes up, 'No, no, Measle can't just give away her daughter. That's not right,' they say.

The tomboy disappears and the abuser flies over the stage laughing malignantly, actually sounding a bit like the tomboy. He swoops down over the helpless Measle and the toddler, who wail noisily. Miss Pie tries to get rid of him, flapping her floury apron at him. When the tomboy returns, there is more pressure from Measle and the tomboy for Miss Pie to take the toddler. Again the Chorus objects.

'Make Measle and the toddler safe,' they suggest, 'and then find out what the abuser's story is.'

This idea baffles Susan. It's not part of her idea of the script, but she concedes, taking Measle and the toddler off the stage and securing them safely in their shoe box home.

'Now let Miss Pie talk to the abuser,' the Chorus demands.

The abuser and the tomboy are on the stage now with Miss Pie. Susan seems baffled, what will happen now? Miss Pie introduces herself to the red-faced abuser who attempts to laugh rudely but actually sounds nervous.

'Ask him what he wants with the toddler,' the Chorus advises.

Gradually, the abuser comes to admit that he needs the toddler to feel complete, that he's nothing without her. He admits and seems to understand that he is hurting the toddler, but he really needs her, he reasserts. The Chorus suggests therapy and the curtain comes down.

We can see from this drama that, as puppeteer, Susan recreated the toddler's abuse, giving her to the abuser and then asking others to intervene. The tomboy and Measle struggle with each other, Measle crying, guilty and helpless, sounding like the toddler, while the tomboy rages on in a manner similar to the abuser. Susan asked that my puppet enter this conflict, and save the toddler from the abuser, angry with this ineffectual baker of pies, and angry with me for not letting her be the co-leader. Both puppet and puppeteer were placed in the bad half of the split world view. The Chorus served to dilute the transference. It broadened the focus of Susan's anger, changed Susan's set script, and forced her to examine why she was doing what she was doing. Neither Miss Pie nor I could have done such a thing, having been banished to a kind of transferential darkness. Anything we could say would have sounded like struggling to get back into the light and would have proved to Susan that we belonged in the darkness. The Chorus served as an

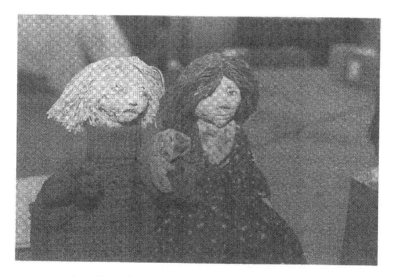

Figure 5.4 The toddler and Miss Pie

impartial witness, wise and all-seeing. 'Make the puppets safe and find out the abuser's story,' it insisted. Of course. Why didn't I think of that?

Just as I couldn't really get into Susan's object world and make changes in there for her, so too, the group pointed out, my puppet couldn't really come between her various puppets. Susan would have to make a choice. If she wanted to continue growing and learning in the group she would have to give up this fossilized drama. She would have to create her own solutions, give the tomboy or Measle the strength and compassion to take the toddler away from the abuser themselves and perhaps help the abuser see that he is not dependent upon this child for his identity. Another option for Susan would be to leave the group for a time to process this material on her own. What was not an option, once everyone could see this dynamic played out, was for her to remain in the group to create and recreate this story. Susan chose to leave the group in order to process the material.

Her leaving the group made it possible for Crystal to enter. Crystal's focus was a little different. She went right to work creating a prince and princess from a far-off planet. Over time she became very enthusiastic about the medium. Within the group she would describe all that she was going to do outside of the group with puppets – form a company with a girlfriend and they would make puppets and go around to hospitals and old folks' homes and there was even mention of television. This focus on Crystal's activities outside of the group and outside of the center was disruptive to the group process. If we tried to pick up a storyline from other puppets, an enticing story would emerge and the focus would magically be back on Crystal. Eventually, my attempts to refocus landed me in the transferential darkness. Crystal began to take group members aside and form alliances and subgroups outside of the group. When the group members realized that what subgrouping was doing to Puppetland, they called a halt to it. Crystal perceived a choice; use the metaphoric language of the group and be a group member, or leave the group. She chose to leave. After she left I asked the group what had happened. They started to talk about backbiting and gossip. I asked if the story could be told in the language of Puppetland. This was the result:

> Once upon a time, a prince and princess from the far-off planet of Xena came to Puppetland. They were shape-shifters and they knew how to appear beautiful in the eyes of all the puppets. But in their hearts they wanted one thing, and that was power. To gain this power they vowed to find the puppets' weakness. They discovered the abyss below

Puppetland, a place filled with darkness and things toxic to puppets. They found a crevice and a way in to the abyss. They then began to feed the toxins to the puppets in unhealthy, tempting, sugary confections. The puppets grew weak and helpless, but never thought to connect their growing helplessness with the toxic confections. One puppet, though, remembered another time in her life when she'd been fed something similar. She stopped eating the stuff and felt better. Then she began to suggest to the other puppets that they not eat the confection and see if it made a difference in how they felt. It did, and together they told the prince and princess from Xena that they should return to their own planet. Artemis, a puppet of the forest, was concerned about this abyss beneath Puppetland. Shouldn't a search party be formed to examine the darkness? Shouldn't some of us climb down and figure out what the toxin is and counter it with something?

'No, no, not today Artemis. We are tired and we need to rest,' said the Chorus.

In this chapter we saw how transference and projection can work, how Susan and Crystal had world views that divided people into good and bad, depending on how powerful they were perceived to be, or on what attention, approval or merging they would be able to provide. We saw how well the group functioned as a Greek Chorus, reminding us of what is and isn't possible for puppets. The group broadened Susan and Crystal's focus so that they were able to see their own dramas with a little more distance; their transference to the group leader was diluted in the process.

Susan made good use of the insights gained during the session described. She moved out of her father's house and got him to agree to attend family therapy. Crystal, however, retreated from the puppetry group and continued to play out her story in other groups.

The patients were too tired at this point to examine the darkness of the abyss, but in the next chapter we will hear and learn the story of smaller and more manageable forms of the abyss: Margaret, the puppet based on Jenny's mother, and the Monster, a puppet created especially for the group to be a player in a winter solstice celebration.

CHAPTER 6

Healing the Split

Margaret, Winter Solstice and the Monster

The first opportunity the group got at working on their individual split-off shadow aspects was provided by Margaret. Margaret, the puppet representing Jenny's mother, or her internalization of the negative aspects of her mother, was well known to the group. They were used to her harsh judgements, her cruel words and her strange living arrangement. The fact that she needed a keeper to keep her safe from the other puppets and to keep them safe from her seemed to be perfectly acceptable, since many of them wished that their own mothers had similar living arrangements. It was actually a rare occasion that we saw her, since Jenny found her so unpleasant to work with. I would preface what follows with the assurance that I don't usually suggest to a patient which puppet they might need to work with, but because this week was different I tried leaving a visual cue which Jenny would be able to use or not as she chose.

> This week of the beginning of Margaret's redemption was a special week. The center was full of the talk of the Lisa Steinberg case, a case of child abuse, spousal abuse and murder within a wealthy lawyer's home in Greenwich Village, Manhattan. Jenny had been talking of nothing else in her groups. Suspecting that there was something about the case that needed working with at a metaphoric level, I came down to the art room ahead of the group and pulled out Margaret and a baby puppet (this was a generic baby that any group member could use) to see what might happen. The rest of the staff arrived, a drama therapist and two interns, and then the patients. Jenny immediately picked up Margaret and began to speak for her. Margaret began saying the most provocative things about how child abuse is justified when you have a brat. The group sat silently, horrified. At this point Alexander walked in, oblivious to the

tone of the group, being in very high spirits and wanting to let Rigvan out of his box to play. Rigvan burst into the group stillness and horror with a little Cossack jig and complimented all the puppets, how fine they all looked today, and then proceeded to tell everyone that he'd made a killing on Wall Street the day before and had been celebrating all night, a thinly veiled reference to Alexander's own drinking. (Puppetry was the only group where Alexander would participate in a discussion of alcoholism, because it was possible for him to speak in terms of Rigvan's drinking and his concern about missing his son's childhood through drink.) Then Alexander looked around and noticed that everyone was sitting in stunned silence.

'What's going on?' he asked.

Jenny very quickly explained that Margaret was just talking about how child abuse is okay when brats were concerned. Alexander pulled back into himself a bit, as if the wind had gone out of a sail.

'Oh my God, and you wonder why I drink. This is why I drink,' Rigvan stated with emphasis. I immediately objected, suggesting that if Rigvan went running for a bottle every time he heard something he didn't like he might end up with a big problem.

But then wanting to keep the discussion at the metaphoric level, I picked up the baby puppet. 'Am I a brat?' Baby asked Margaret.

'Yes, of course you are and you are homely, too,' said Margaret.

'Awwwww,' wailed Baby and now the group members found their voices. The Greek Chorus had returned.

'No, Margaret,' they objected, 'you can't talk to a baby that way. Try it again.' After several attempts to say something nice to Baby, Margaret gave up.

'What's wrong with you that you can't say something nice to the baby?' asked Rigvan.

'I have a devil in me,' said Margaret, 'a child-abuse devil.'

'Let's kill her,' Rigvan suggested to the other puppets.

'Oh no,' said Ungar, 'you can't kill her, that would release the child-abuse devil among us.'

'No, no we don't want that,' begged the Chorus.

'Well, will she change her ways?' asked Rigvan.

'No,' Margaret stated defiantly.

'How did you come to have a child-abuse devil in you?' I asked Margaret.

'I was a brat and my mother abused me,' she replied quietly. At this point Rigvan, who had been creeping up on Margaret with a weapon of some kind (a ballpoint pen) pulled back. Alexander rubbed his head and Rigvan said, 'I don't feel very well in my head.'

'Did you deserve to be abused?' I asked.

'Yes, of course, I was a brat,' Margaret said with satisfaction. (She had been 'in control' of the abuse, she had caused her mother to abuse her by being a brat.)

'Well then, we need to have a ceremony,' suggested the drama therapist. 'Margaret, today is the last day of your old life and the first day of your new life. You need to get into the basket. (Conveniently the baby puppet had a perfect-sized bassinet/basket.) Jenny carefully placed Margaret in the basket. 'Now everyone will give you a gift on this special day, starting with Baby.' The basket was then sent over to me.

Looking down at this bad mother from the point of view of the abused baby was a powerfully uncomfortable experience. I was barely able to croak out an 'I wish you wisdom' before quickly passing the puppet to the drama therapy intern.

Ungar looked down on Margaret, calling up every shamanic, tribal memory he could find. 'I bid the devil in you be transformed on this day.' The tone was set, the instructions were clear. Each group member would get a chance to look at, confront and give a gift to Margaret. Their internalized bad objects, which they would have projected onto Margaret, would receive the gift.

The next patient was too angry with her own mother to be interested in anything but destroying Margaret, so after glaring at the puppet in the basket, she passed it on to the next patient.

This next patient's mother, a holocaust survivor, had killed herself when her oldest son, the patient, confronted her abuse of narcotics. He had never been able to resolve that relationship, never been able to express his sorrow for having hurt or shamed her. He felt as though she had taken that from him by killing herself. His puppet looked down on Margaret and spoke with a certain harshness, pulling away from her as he spoke. 'You better change your ways, because if you don't we'll take away the baby, we'll raise it ourselves, we could do that, and we would cut out your tongue.'

The next patient's puppet moved in closer and said, 'The gift I give you is the gift of love. I don't think you got enough love growing up, so that's my gift to you.' And saying that the little puppet leaned into the basket and gave Margaret a kiss. At this point Jenny began crying quietly to herself.

Alexander took the basket and Rigvan began speaking with his Ukrainian accent, very serious now, no joking around about wanting to murder her. He told her that he loved her but that she couldn't abuse her child. It was not allowed. As he talked he became more serious, putting his puppet down, simply talking directly to Margaret. He assured her that if she abused the child one more time, the child would be taken away from her and she would never see her child again, ever. (In actuality Alexander had said something very similar the last time he was with his own mother. He had refused, after that meeting, to have any contact with her.) Again he reassured her that he loved her and that he prayed she get the help she needed so that she could keep her baby and then passed her to the drama therapist.

The drama therapist let her little blue dog lick Margaret's face and promise to come visit and share Chinese take-out, especially ribs. At this Jenny was chuckling through her tears. Then the drama therapist passed the basket to her and told her to take Margaret out. That today was a new day for her.

Jenny put Margaret on, still fighting tears. She promised that she would work with Eric, the psychiatrist puppet, twice a week now. She knew there were other things a person could do instead of being mean to your kids when you feel bad. She could call a friend, or punch a pillow. She would practice being good to the baby puppet.

'Can you give the baby a hug?' asked the drama therapist.

So Margaret and the baby hugged and the group sighed. Margaret and all of the internalized bad mothers were on the road to reconciliation. Everyone sat quietly for a moment and then Alexander looked at his watch. The drama therapist noted that he'd worked very hard and that in the business of helping someone else to heal perhaps one heals oneself as well. 'We should let Rigvan have the last word,' she added.

Rigvan looked around at the other puppets and said he knew about suffering and abuse, that life had been very hard in the Gulags. 'You deserve good lives, all of you,' he said quietly, but with real feeling. 'God bless you. I love you all.' And then he tried to do a little jig but groaned and laughed. Everyone smiled and returned his blessing.

This was a very moving session for everyone in the room but most of all for Jenny and for Alexander. When Alexander said that he prayed Margaret get the help she needed so that she could keep her baby, this was an expression of reconciliation towards his own internalized mother. He had not been able to say anything as conciliatory or hopeful to his actual mother, but Margaret provided him with an opportunity to verbalize the wish. It wasn't his actual mother that he carried around in his mind, but rather an image of how she had been, a fossilized, one-dimensional memory that influenced his thinking and his decisions. It was carrying around this internalized bad mother that caused him to see the world from the victim point of view. This day, however, saw a lessening of the hold that internalized object had on him. After that session Alexander repeatedly requested to review the videotape of the session, looking at the whole experience from the distance and objectivity that time and the video provide, further lessening the hold of his inner bad mother.

For Jenny, the session was also extremely powerful. When Margaret was passed from person to person, we observed Jenny's mood change. She was strongly identified with Margaret, belligerent and remorseless at first. As patients struggled to verbalize their wishes for Margaret, Jenny began to empathize with the child and the mother. When the one puppet leaned in and said he would give her love and then kissed her, Jenny's sorrow became evident. She had not often been freely offered love in her life. As we saw in Chapter 3, this was not something she was comfortable with. By the time Margaret came back to Jenny, the rigidity about Margaret's belligerence and remorselessness was gone. Margaret couldn't help but hear and take in all that the other puppets had said to her. She expressed Jenny's wish to begin to heal some of the anguish in the relationship with the baby, to begin to talk over these things with Eric more often, to ask for the help that would keep her connected with the baby and with the community.

This relationship with the community was key in Margaret's beginning to find 'redemption'. We saw the group taking on the role of the Greek Chorus with Susan and again in this session. Both Susan and Jenny came to the point where they would have to allow their puppets to change in order to remain a part of the group. Susan decided to take her internalized objects away, keep them from interacting with the group and being changed by that interaction. Jenny decided to allow Margaret to stay and begin to be reconciled with her other puppets and with the various puppets in the group.

Robert Bly (1988) wrote about the shadow parts of the self, not as necessarily negative but as being everything about us that is not conscious, the Jungian personal unconscious. He envisioned a bag, 'the long bag we drag behind us', filled with things we are not conscious of, or things we want to repress. I see Bly's long bag, a wonderful metaphor in itself, as being full of potential puppets, little images of people or parts of the self. When a person creates a puppet, projecting internalized objects onto the puppet, that image or part of the self is taken out of the bag, out of the darkness and shadow. By changing it from an image in darkness to a fully realized, three-dimensional image something is changed. By interacting with others more change occurs. If a person leaves the part of the self in the bag, they can stay safe, little fossilized objects that are completely predictable. Initially, Susan's internalized abuser was returned to the bag, where he could continue to cause her misery in a predictable way. Some choose the misery that is known over the discomfort of the unknown and unpredictable. Jenny took Margaret out of the bag and brought her into the light of consciousness, the group's and her own. From each exchange with the puppets in the group Margaret received a gift and with each gift she and Jenny were irrevocably changed.

Although the session with Margaret had moved most of the group further on the path of integrating their various split-off 'bad mothers', there still seemed to be more work to be done. A collective shadow, the abyss below Puppetland, filled with 'toxic' and unknown things, had yet to be explored. Could a puppet be created that would embody some of the fear and darkness of the abyss? Could it be 'dark' enough to be a real representation and yet small enough to work with and not be overwhelming? To that end the Monster was created. The Monster was a ragged brown and black creature that looked like it just crawled out of the abyss. He was created to play the role of the group shadow in the Jungian sense, but literally as well in our winter solstice celebration.

The Christmas, Chanukkah, New Year's season was always a difficult one. Some time before Thanksgiving many of the patients would begin to recall their worst memories of the season and the stories and misery would build up to the climax of New Year's Eve. For some there was a sense of defeat in facing the new year and still being held captive by symptoms or even by the mental health system.

To counter this loss of community that the holiday blues fostered, we planned a non-sectarian celebration marking the longest night of the year and the return of the light. The group began working on a mural of the Wise Old Woman's hearth and yule tree with lots of gifts under it (Figure 6.1). A table was filled with a feast and logs blazed in the fireplace. Patients who weren't part of the puppetry group watched the work progressing with interest and two individuals asked if they could help, adding a braided rag rug for the floor and a swag of holly for the mantle.

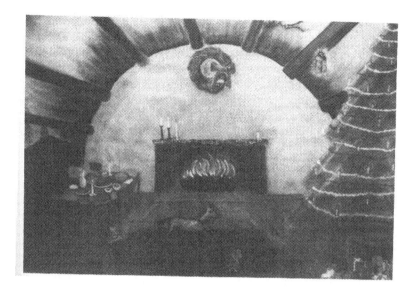

Figure 6.1 The Wise Old Woman's hearth

A simple Chinese dragon puppet, brightly colored to scare off the darkness, was created out of long sheets of paper attached to dowels. Several puppets manipulated it, each holding up his own dowel and part of the dragon, a kind of puppet's puppet. Bells and candles were collected to ensure that light would prevail over darkness.

Various group members promised to bring in food and juice or soda so that the puppeteers could celebrate as well. The day of the party arrived. A tape of Paul Winter's music played in the background and the Monster entered, representing the fear and the darkness that the group wanted to banish. He growled noisily and the puppets picked up the dragon and bells and chased the Monster around the art room and into a supply closet, a mysterious closet that had another door which connected to the theater. This seemed the perfect place for the Monster to live.

Then candles were lit and food was brought out. The mural graced one end of the table. It was a truly delightful celebration, filled with feelings of generosity and joy. Toasts were made to good friends present and those who were no longer there. Hopes were expressed for a good new year filled with many blessings. A new group member, deeply touched by all of the good feeling, expressed his warmth and surprise at being included and at feeling a part of the celebration. He said that this was not something that happened to him. Even if he were included in things, which was rare, he would not feel a part of it, never having learned how to be with other people. So he thanked everyone for whatever magic was involved and they toasted him and hoped he would stay in the group.

All of this was wonderful in its own right, but the thing that happened because of the celebration was that the group became interested in what happened to the Monster. During subsequent sessions questions emerged. Where had he really gone? Who was he really? Was he always a monster? Why didn't the group know about him sooner? Could they meet him again and ask him their questions himself? Why not?

And so it was that the Monster became a part of the group. And this is how the story was handed down over time.

This is the tale of the Monster and his three sons, High, Medium and Low. The Monster was first seen during a bleak and dreary winter. He was a great, hairy, unknown, frightening creature that lurked near the edge of the forest during a winter solstice celebration. It happened that the puppets had been feeling the darkness as a great weight on their hearts and the Wise Old Woman knew what was called for was a ceremony to bring back the light. When the puppets caught sight of this shadowy figure lurking they felt it was the realization of their fear and they wanted to chase it from Puppetland. With great noise and firelight they did chase the Monster deeper into the forest. They felt the heaviness lift from their hearts as they bid the Monster and the darkest night farewell.

Now it happened that Carey, a puppet given to rather monstrous moods herself, was wandering deep within the woods one day and throwing rocks at trees. She took great satisfaction at the sound that the rock made as it thunked against a tree. Well, she would throw and hear the thunk and smile to herself and then throw some more, but then she heard instead of the one thunk there were two thunks. How could that be? She looked all around and sure enough she was not alone. The Monster was there with her. Now she got a good look at him, which in the flurry of the celebration she hadn't been able to do to her satisfaction. He was indeed hairy and ragged and his eyes looked like limpid pools of toxic waste and he smelled bad. Most puppets would have immediately run but there was a certain strength about Carey, being the daughter of

Margaret, that was not put off by much of anything, especially not monsters. So they began to throw rocks together and soon they were having a contest. They were evenly matched and they fairly wore themselves out so they sat down together and the Monster told Carey his story in a series of rude and disgusting noises, which, surprisingly, she felt she recognized. His language seemed to be made up of a series of grunts and coughs and gags that resonated somewhere in Carey's memory. Carey understood. He told her that although he had always looked this way and perhaps never learned the human puppet art of hygiene, he had only begun really to feel monstrous around the time that his wife left him to care for his three sons. They were growing boys and he really didn't know much about caring for himself, let alone three monster boys. They were so demanding and High was getting as big as a tree. What was a monster to do? He showed her his heart which was usually hidden, and she could see there was a crack in it and flames around it.

Carey was deeply sympathetic. She revealed the Monster's sad tale to the rest of Puppetland and they, too, understood. They agreed not to chase him around with bells and candles and dragons any more, but they couldn't quite bring themselves to get too close to him for all the bad smells and rude noises. It must be admitted here that of all the puppets in Puppetland, Carey was the most tolerant in that regard.

The story of the Monster emerged in a session sometime following the winter solstice party. Alexander began playing the Monster and Jenny, using her Carey puppet, spontaneously began to play with him and translate his grunts and snorts. The group sat quietly, listening to the story, nodding at his reasons for feeling monstrous and laughing and groaning at all of his disgusting, asocial ways. Eventually, a full body puppet had to be created to represent High and two baby monsters were created representing Medium and Low, in order to more fully integrate the Monster and his narrative into the group history. They continued to live together in the mysterious forest of the supply closet, not willing to undergo the rigors of hygiene and polite conversation that civilization would require of them. The Monster was the quintessential wild man that Bly (1988) described as coming out of the pond in the Grimm brothers' story of 'Iron John'. This wild man was neither a tame, obedient man, nor a violent, savage man, but something in between. Bly wrote of the story of the wild man allowing shadow material to be reintegrated slowly in a way that doesn't overwhelm or damage the ego. He felt the encounter with the wild man was about play rather than fighting (p.53).

The Monster, like the wild man, allowed the group to approach their collective shadow in a playful way. They made him welcome and a part of the whole, integrating him into the history of Puppetland and yet acknowledging his need to live in the forest in his own way. They could be with him in the light of day, explore his story, want to learn more about his children, but give him a respectful distance. They did not feel a fear of being killed or abused by him or the need to kill him off, nor did they repress him, or stuff him back into the bag. He remained there, living in his forest with his three sons, coming out from time to time to see how the world was progressing.

CHAPTER 7

Reparation and the
Wise Old Woman
The Conclusion

Loss and reparation

An aspect of working in a large day treatment facility in New York City was the turnover rate among the staff. Roughly half the staff were students and when the school year came to an end we would all have to deal with termination. Puppetry had its own way of integrating the loss. We could use ceremony, group mourning and reparation and all of it could occur on the mythic plane, taking it out of the everyday reality and perhaps even heightening the experience. One example was the loss of Ungar, the puppet, and of course the puppeteer, LeClanche Du Rand. At the end of her internship, Du Rand was able to explain that her internship was over and then was able to enact the process of termination through the puppet, telling how Ungar had to move on, that he had to find his own tribe now. This was something the group could work with creatively. Alexander, having grown quite attached over the year, was able to use Rigvan to express his sorrow to Ungar. The feelings were real and they were expressed, probably more easily, in this metaphoric form. This is how the story was told.

> Soon it was time for Rigvan's great friend, Ungar, to move on. He felt his own tribe and family must be just beyond the horizon and he knew he must go in search of them. So he prepared to set out to find them, gathering his few belongings and many memories. At the feast given in honor of the time they had spent together and the learning they had all shared, Ungar told this story.

He had gone for a walk in the forest on Rigvan's estate, where they had spent many fine hours hunting and riding together. Ungar was feeling unsure and distraught over the calling he heard in his heart to find his own family because it would mean leaving this tribe he had grown to love. While in the forest he ran across a Wise Old Woman who had been there for more than one hundred years. Up until then none of the puppets realized that she lived in the forest. She seemed like the kindest and wisest person he had ever met, so he told her his story, his love for the tribe, but the calling in his heart. The Wise Old Woman, the keeper of secrets and herbs, a healer and a great-grandmother to many, had lived a long life and knew about callings and losses and even about sorrows. She said that he would need a talisman, a 'guide' to help him through the loss and to help him keep to his path. She said that the other members of the tribe would each need a talisman as well. She gave Ungar little beads made of baked earth each with a face on it, one for each puppet to help each find his or her true path and to remind them of their dear friend Ungar. When he had finished the telling he went around to each puppet and gave each a talisman. So amid much feasting and songs and speeches, Rigvan and the rest of the puppets bid farewell to Ungar and wished him Godspeed. And later they would reminisce, telling of the Great Hunt, the day that Vedrina arrived and Victoria and Rigvan did not fight to the death.

It seemed that Du Rand had planted in the community mind a group myth. Although we were losing her and her puppet, there was this gift, this archetypal Wise Old Woman that had come to life in story. Some time went by and it became clear that perhaps the group could benefit by the addition of this character, a nurturing, caring elder, in puppet form. To that end I created the Wise Old Woman. Once she was finished, she was brought to life by the group as a whole. Each member had a chance to hold her or work her and to listen for something about who she was and what gift she had to give to the individual. We all listened carefully as the puppet was passed around and in this way she developed a kind of group character, accepting the projections of each of our internalized good objects (Figure 7.1).

From these projections we learned that she had gifts for each of us, that she was 104 and that she lived in an underground hogan, or kiva. The Hopi use their kivas for secret religious ritual, so by giving her this kind of dwelling she was given spiritual associations as well. It was also discovered that she had Native American blood (giving her more of a sense of place and belonging than the rest of the puppets or puppeteers had previously felt

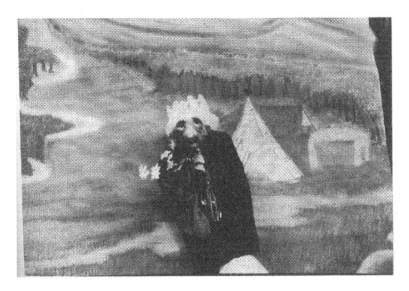

Figure 7.1 The Wise Old Woman

about themselves) and that she had knowledge of the earth, its herbs, seasons, and life. All of the projections were warm and generous. There was no horror, no negative projection, a surprising thing since nearly all of the puppeteers had histories of trauma and abuse and seemed to have an easier time recalling negative projections than positive. But it was apparent that this puppet tapped some vestigial memories of positive, comforting caregiving. It didn't take long for her home to become a gathering place, like the ceilidh houses of Ireland and Scotland, where the tribe could share stories, food and dreams around her hearth.

From the Wise Old Woman's emergence I learned something about the importance of generosity and the possibility of creative reparation around the wrenching and rupture that loss necessitates. For all of us, she was a generous character, we projected generosity onto her and then reintegrated it, as seen in the group mural of her home for the winter solstice celebration (see Figure 6.1). In the previous chapter, we saw how when others outside of the puppet-making group viewed the mural and asked for the story behind the picture, they also became interested in adding something to the work, in expressing something generous. It seemed these small acts of generosity did much to repair the sense of loss that the holidays always brought.

The Wise Old Woman taught us the importance of accepting loss, but also that along with the acceptance was the possibility of creative reparation. This emerged many times, but one of the clearest examples was when Alexander sent his puppet Rigvan to the spas of Europe to 'dry out'. The final and favorite in his tours of European spas was in a place called Split. I think he was making an effort to heal his internal splits (thus the choice of the name) but it meant a loss, a giving up of old habits and ways of seeing. We have all experienced or observed resistance: whenever something is to be given up there is a matching wish to maintain things just as they are. Being creatures of habit we are often fearful of change. But again the Wise Old Woman came forward with words of comfort.

> After Rigvan's return from Europe it seemed that his soul was at peace with itself. How was he to maintain and even carry this peace forward? He consulted the Wise Old Woman who reminded him of the wisdom of the sweat lodge, long walks and storytelling with his family around the fire in the evenings. The Wise Old Woman also told him that horror and helplessness at different points in a puppet's life makes the puppet strong and compassionate, that it can be seen as a rite of passage through which a puppet joins the rest of puppetkind and learns to care more for others, that relationships grow deeper and stronger. Rigvan nodded, knowing she spoke the truth. They found a great friendship and he and his family became a comfort to her in the winter of her years. (On her 104th birthday she had decided the rest of her years would simply be the 'winter years'.)

Later, having learned a great deal from this group projection, I felt a need to create my own puppet, an apprentice to live in the forest, not yet wise enough to live underground, but willing to learn about herbs and healing hearts. We were having yet another gathering at the end of another intern's time at our center, sitting around the art room table which had so often become the transitional space of Puppetland. I asked the puppets to make a list of things they felt they were holding on to and things they felt that they could let go of. A list of the puppets' concerns would be more accessible than individual concerns hidden under layers of resistance and denial. Most of the lists of things being held on to included fears, emptiness, sadness, reality, despair. Most of the lists of things that could be let go of included these same things. My concern, through the apprentice, was fear of loss of the Wise Old Woman. Loss was prominent in my mind, now that the intern was leaving. I had begun to contemplate the idea of finishing a dissertation started what seemed like a lifetime ago. I was concerned about having to devote time and attention to a dissertation and not being able to work at the center any more. So Artemis wrote that she was fearful of losing the Wise Old Woman and yet the thing she needed to let go of was the Wise Old Woman. I then asked everyone to turn the paper over and to write down a gift for their puppet, the thing they needed most. Some of the gifts were abstract things like happiness, friendship and feeling whole. Most were concrete things that would bring the puppet (or puppeteer) happiness: art, maps, dance classes, a ride on the Central Park carousel, a sapling, a peppermint stick, art supplies and three wishes for friends. What I wrote as a gift for Artemis was compassion; if she was to become the Wise Old Woman one day, she would need strength, wisdom and compassion to be true to herself.

I think Artemis represented all of us. She was facing the loss of the Wise Old Woman, much as we all were facing the loss of the intern and the eventual loss of the group. We all needed strength, wisdom and compassion to be true to ourselves, like Ungar's talismans and 'guides' for our separate journeys. When the task was done, Alexander asked if he could read the lists and the gifts to the group, without giving the name of the puppet. The group agreed to this suggestion, eager to hear what everyone else had written. When I picked up the pieces of paper after the group was over I saw he had added additional gifts to all the sheets of paper. He had not read these additions, he was not looking for acknowledgement of what he had done. They were simply his wishes for the puppet and the puppeteer, and in each case they were strong, wise and compassionate gifts.

Of all the kinds of groups I ran at the center (art, pottery, verbal groups, film or volleyball) I never found such acts of generosity, such joy as I found in this group. I suspected, at the end of this session, that all would be well, that we had the tools or 'guides' we needed to carry on.

Conclusions

While the first part of the book dealt with Jenny's struggle and resolution of early childhood trauma, the last part examined the healing that occurred at the group level where patients created story and puppets. We examined reparation that occurred in the creation of narratives and metaphors. We saw how a stable community was created, with a sense of history, by a population better known for instability and a dissociated sense of history.

Looking back over the work done at the center with these individuals, I see that the patients had created defensive stances that made a great deal of sense, given the trauma that was inflicted on them. From observation, I saw art as therapeutic for the patient in and of itself, that the creative process unlocked the possibility for the sense of self to achieve new levels of integration and growth, free of the defensive stance. Patients entered puppetry with internalized objects, both good and bad. They projected them onto puppets of their own creation, much as they might project onto the therapist or mother in projective identification. These puppets with all the narratives and attached metaphors of growth and change would then be internalized and carried around like transitional objects, things of their own making that made them feel whole and happy, not alienated, not dissociated.

I saw the role of the art therapist as the support of the patient's creative efforts, as an ally to the creative aspect of the self, and that it was the patient's own work that had the ameliorative effect on the rest of the aspects of the self.

The conclusions I draw from this work are that trauma and abuse of a child create a developmental rupture in the individual's sense of self, which leads to many symptoms and a variety of diagnoses. Not only can we observe this rupture within the artistic expressions of self, in art therapy, but we also observe that the creative process can be used to repair the disturbed body image, the dissociated sense of self, the disjointed sense of history and causality, as well as the feeling of alienation from self and other.

Perhaps a generally accepted view in the field of art therapy is that puppets are the exclusive domain of drama therapists and children. I would like to challenge that view by emphasizing the fundamental importance of body image development and representation in art therapy. Edith Kramer taught us to provide the patient with the tools to sublimate unacceptable drives. I found that many of this group of patients seemed too scattered, too unfocused, too dissociated to sublimate. I felt compelled to go back further in human development, where I found indications that before being able to sublimate the individual needs to have a cohesive sense of self. Humans need an integrated body image. As art therapists we can help our patients develop a stronger sense of being in the world, which seems especially necessary when working with patients whose bodies and sense of being were violated at an early age. From working repeatedly and in a playful way with representations of body image, it was possible to externalize this felt sense of being in the world. The careful attention to a body image representation creates a parallel internal sense of care. These patients may not have experienced a level of physical care to their bodies; they may, in fact, have internalized many negative things from their trauma experiences. Working with body image over time is a way to help transform these feelings into positive experiences. I believe only after establishing a stable sense of being in the world can individuals use art therapy for sublimation. Finally, puppet making may be a very skillful way for adults to work with body image representations to bring about these positive changes for themselves, and in that it is certainly not just the domain of drama therapists or children.

CHAPTER 8

Postscript
Tying Up Loose Ends

Notes on Jenny's life after spring 1988

At this point I should include a note on how Jenny's story continued after the year documented. Our interviews were finished and Jenny began working on writing her autobiography for herself rather than giving me her lengthy journal entries. She continued in her art groups, puppetry and pottery. In puppetry she was finally able to confront Margaret (the puppet) and in the process seemed to clearly understand just how damaged Margaret (her mother) had been through her own history of abuse.

In 1991 Jenny again got a new counselor and in 1993 began to separate from the center, setting up an arts and crafts studio in the housing project where she and Sally lived. It had a working kiln and she had a budget and was able to take on the role of 'the art lady' for the residents. But it seemed that there was psychological payment to be made for this move towards independence. Jenny fell on a wet floor in her lobby and broke her ankle. Due to her weight and perhaps psychological factors her physical rehabilitation was unsuccessful, resulting in the confirmation of her earlier fears and fantasies of being confined to a wheelchair for the rest of her life.

She chose not to return to the center because wheelchair access was less than convenient and because she was moving towards independence. She continued to see one of the music therapists from the other center privately for a while, and won large settlements from several lawsuits, including for the wet lobby of a city-owned housing project. She also explained to me that she had started up a home nursing service, because she knew what patients needed and could work as a kind of go-between, healing any splits or rifts that might occur between patient and nurse. She described this as very satisfying.

Her mother, Margaret, died in early 1995, but before she died Jenny was able to ask her questions about why she let Jenny be abused by her uncle and brother. She questioned Margaret about this and other vague recollections and was actually glad to have them confirmed for her. Margaret then told Jenny she was truly sorry for everything that had happened to her and 'cried for three days and then had a stroke and died' (Gerity 1997, p.96). At last contact, Jenny seemed to be feeling optimistic, somewhat liberated, reporting that she was looking for a literary agent to whom she could sell her memoirs.

A note on other puppeteers

The puppeteers who have contacted me since my departure from the center are doing well, returning perhaps gingerly to their professional lives or training programs and further education. They get together from time to time and remember the group with fondness, reviewing the old stories and myths that had touched them and even bringing out one of the old puppets upon occasion.

Notes on the inclusion of culture and ethnicity

As I was reviewing Jenny's case, the thought occurred to me that if I had used the internalized image or representation of the fondly remembered great-grandmother, a lot of the developmental process might have been facilitated more easily and perhaps even more quickly. It seemed that I worked very hard to help her internalize good experiences and positive feelings, ignoring the obvious fact that she had an internalized good object of her own cultural and racial background and one that would have come from her own personal history. Sweet Basil, the doll I had made, was introduced as a transitional object to comfort Jenny while I was at a conference and she developed into something more because of Jenny's needs. I think it was a wonderful intervention that I stumbled my way into, but I think Jenny was leaving clues that she would have liked to work with a representation of her great-grandmother as well, clues which I didn't see until much later.

I can imagine what progress might have been made if Jenny had created a great-grandmother doll that would have helped Sweet Basil care for Little Jenny, Little Joy and Little Carey. I can imagine all kinds of possibilities for more little quilts and maybe even the big one that her mother never made for her. As I reread the interviews I could imagine what a delightful, empowering experience it would have been to interview this positive matriarch from Jenny's own history.

Perhaps by including this concept in the book, I am leaving the reader with the idea of a group of Wise Old Women living in a forest who come from a variety of cultural or ethnic backgrounds, much as Du Rand left the puppet group with an image of a kindly, wise elder when she was terminating.

If I am ever in the position to work with individuals who have different backgrounds from my own, I would be sure not to miss the opportunity to help the patient develop a positive object of their own background. I suspect I missed this one because I enjoyed Jenny's relationship with Sweet Basil and felt almost as if I were able to be a part of the internalization process. I could certainly see the positive effect of creating a transitional object for her and I suspect I may not have wanted to relinquish Sweet Basil's importance in her life. I am sure this is a piece of my own countertransference, which I will now explain.

Countertransference

At its deepest layer of countertransference, this case was greatly influenced by events in my personal life. In the spring of 1988 I learned that my husband was terminally ill. I believe my reluctance to relinquish Sweet Basil's importance in Jenny's life was a reflection of other things I was reluctant to relinquish. Along with this reluctance on my part was a reaching towards an understanding of abandonment depression, internalization of good objects, object constancy, representations of self and other, whole object relations as well as the importance of mourning something or someone that is lost to you. In reviewing this material, years later, I can see that my life situation had an impact on the case.

Treatment under these conditions was difficult and my life circumstance necessitated that I withdraw some of my energy from work that spring. This coincided, fortunately, with Jenny's growing strength and independence. In retrospect it would also seem that Jenny benefited from my struggles to integrate the impending loss as well as the struggles to make reparations.

At a less personal level there was everyday transference and counter-transference that occurred because I was the provider of materials and space for creative expression. The creative arts therapies could function without the invasive qualities that patients perceived in verbal therapies. In addition, the art room, pottery room and myself were all seen as fixtures, to the point that we achieved a certain level of object constancy which counselors rarely achieved because most of them left after a year or two.

Utilizing early defenses, the abuse survivor tended to split. Here was a perfect opportunity for splitting. The counselors made them feel uncomfortable, always asking them to talk about things that were unspeakable, but the art therapist gently offered art materials, a way of saying, 'find your own metaphors and images and let *them* speak for you'. The counselors often received rage while the art therapist more often received positive feelings. The counselors and their supervisors began to grow understandably weary of such splitting. They would sometimes find it very difficult to establish a working alliance with these patients. It was much easier for the art therapists to establish alliances with these patients because of the positive transference and countertransference that was usually a part of the art room experience.

A further example of the perils of transference and splitting occurred in Jenny's case because she (as Joy) was receiving music therapy at a separate agency and thus a competition was set up between the 'good' music therapists who treated Joy and the 'good' art therapist who treated Jenny.

It would have served Jenny better if we had communicated on a regular basis, or if the components of Jenny's treatment were at the same center, but transference, splitting and the countertransferential wish to be the only 'good' therapist, the beloved object, got in the way. The seriousness of the split became clear when one of the music therapists, in a moment of exasperation, gave Joy a directive to 'get rid of Jenny'. Her thinking was that Joy should be more consistent with her identity and stop using the name Jenny. In Jenny's literal way of thinking this meant 'killing off', and since she weighed 300 pounds, each personality must weigh 100 pounds. So if she lost 100 pounds then Jenny would be dead. After some bouts of dizziness in various groups, along with excessively bad moods, I asked Jenny what was going on. She explained that she was dieting in order to follow the music therapist's directive. I pointed out to her that she might just lose a little weight in each area of herself and that was the end of trying to 'get rid of Jenny'. I did communicate to the music therapist the result of her directive and she decided not to pursue the issue of 'getting rid of' aspects of Jenny any further, although she believed Joy was the core personality and that these other aspects should not be 'encouraged'. Disaster had been averted, but this basic difference in the way we saw Jenny, or the way Jenny revealed herself to us, unfortunately seemed to block our ability to communicate easily or to coordinate treatment.

Notes on creating an art group for survivors

When the idea of a survivors' art group was first proposed, alarm bells went off in my mind. What would the make up of the group be; would the patients be selected or would it be voluntary? Both men and women expressed interest in the group. Could a group like this be co-educational? Many of our patients had very fragile coping skills, often with histories of self-abusive behavior. How would the decision be made about someone being too fragile for the group? Could a survivors' group aggravate symptoms? Could such a group be re-traumatizing? I was just scared, usually an indication of a good idea in my experience. For these patients safety was a unfamiliar concept. The closest they could come to a concept of safety was an idea of control. If they were in control maybe then they would be safe. The firm belief that someone would always hurt them precluded any possible feelings of safety. How was a therapist to present an alternative experience? It took several months to develop a rhythm that provided the needed safety to allow for the patients to become comfortable enough to simply stay in the group without panic.

There was a natural resistance around the issue of attendance. If one session was extremely meaningful the next week's attendance would be low. It was almost as if the group members couldn't take too much supportive interaction, interaction that went against the world view of a damaged and hurt child. But an interruption in their attendance would interrupt their sense of continuity as a group. One week would be like a new group full of merging and relief at having a place to be understood, and then the next week would be sparsely attended and those who were there seemed embarrassed for what had been revealed the week before. It seemed that the group could never quite move out of the beginning stages.

As a way of dealing with both attendance and crisis management I began to bring in various articles to read while the group members worked on their art. Most material would be from books written for survivors, like *The Courage to Heal* (Bass and Davis 1988) and *Reach for the Rainbow* (Finney 1990). I could go through the table of contents or the index and ask the group what sounded most helpful. This gave them the much-needed feeling of being in control. It would also provide the defense of intellectualization (one of my favorites), some distance from the painful feelings and education about symptoms that they all shared. My reading various materials made dialogue possible. I wasn't the authority, I was looking for answers just as they were. I could present an idea and it could be discussed. The space felt more flexible this way and it worked well. The group members were able to see that they were not alone. The world was not so strictly divided between the child and the demanding, pain-inducing other.

While discussing their artwork as well as the readings, there began to be more of a feeling of continuity. There was no longer the pressure to reveal terrible family secrets, or to re-traumatize themselves in the process. I could ask them what they would like to hear about the following week as a means of providing closure and instilling a sense of future sessions, so that the group could come back and work some more. We didn't have to sort through all of the contents of Pandora's box on that one day, in that 55-minute session. We would come back to anything they needed to come back to. Once they felt safe enough they were able to give each other hugs or small words of comfort as additional closure if a session had been rough.

Some of the material that I brought in suggested working with the inner child. I was aware that the dissociative patients in the group had inner children. I was aware that everyone in the group had a tendency or a capacity to look at the world as if they were wounded children about to be hurt again. I had also read about some of Milton Erickson's work with the unconscious (Erickson and Rossi 1979). He felt that because of the unconscious' lack of awareness of time, the past can be very immediate in one's dreams or in a flashback. The idea of somehow reaching the parts of the individual that had been locked away inside, since these traumas occurred, was intriguing.

In order to address the attendance/resistance issue (and to work with the 'inner child') I suggested that on alternate weeks I bring in some 'lighter' material, fairy tales for example. Everyone approved as they were quite aware of their reluctance to return after a particularly intense session. I dug out my copy of Bruno Bettelheim's *The Uses of Enchantment* (1977), an excellent discussion of the therapeutic value of fairy tales. He explained that by a parent's telling of a fairy tale to the child the feelings evoked by the story were shared. The child could feel understood: 'As he listens, the child feels understood in his most tender longings, his most ardent wishes, his most severe anxieties and feelings of misery, as well as in his highest hopes' (p.154). The tale told can give the child a feeling of not being alone with the darker, more irrational aspects of the self. It can present suggestions on how to deal constructively with these inner experiences. There is a feeling of possibilities and hope that by hard work and clever planning resolutions are possible. 'He senses from fairy tales that to be a human being in this world of ours means to accept difficult challenges, but also encountering wondrous adventures' (p.155).

Having survived many traumas, the group members had many dark, irrational parts; experiences which they had internalized. They had many problems that needed resolution, many anxieties and fears which could be dealt with on the unconscious or preconscious level by the telling of fairy tales. One of the more difficult inner experiences that the group members dealt with was aggression. Some group members, more often the men in the group, freely expressed this inner experience on paper as well as verbally. This was very frightening to some of the others in the group, more often the women who were unwilling to acknowledge their own aggressive feelings but would act them out by hurting themselves.

Displaced aggression was a common phenomenon. Group members might come into the group feeling angry and not knowing why. They might express their aggressive feelings in their artwork or often in attacking the group leader for bringing in the 'wrong' reading material. The other group members might also feel attacked and they would respond with aggression. Any limit setting at this point would be viewed as aggressive as well. Eventually all this aggression would be turned inward, with members toying with suicidal feelings, or acting symbolically by destroying their artwork. Clearly, fairy tales that dealt with aggression were needed.

The tale 'Fitcher's Feathered Bird' from the Brothers Grimm (Segal and Sendak 1973) was one of the first I read to this group. Everyone was delighted and relieved. It had all the necessary elements. There was an evil sorcerer who could catch beautiful girls by assuming the appearance of a poor beggar man and touching the pretty girl's sleeve. The girl then became powerless and would be captured. Everyone in the group could identify with the victim that was powerless to a touch. The story had a key that opened the door to a forbidden room. Everyone knew the strength of temptation of such a key. Another element in this story was dismembered bodies of all the pretty girls that were captured by the evil sorcerer. All of the group members groaned at this as it touched on their issues of body image and dissociation. But there was also the youngest daughter in this story who was very clever and brave. She used the forbidden key and reached right into all the gore until she fished out all the body parts of her sisters. She was able to put them together in the right order which, with her good intentions, brought them back to life. It was the keeping of the parts separate that kept them from being alive. This too was a concept that rang true for the dissociative patients. At the end of the story she saves herself and her sisters by tricking the sorcerer into carrying them home, where she then rolls about in honey and feathers in order to be mistaken for Fitcher's Bird. The brothers come, lock up the sorcerer in his house and burn it down.

This story, with all its gore, horror and revenge, was a delight to the group. Even the anorectics, who didn't believe that aggressive feelings were ever acceptable, applauded the end. It presented their most troubling concerns in a way that could be talked about without being acted out. This story touched on the issues of aggression, revenge fantasies and even childhood pyromania, and it provided a feeling of resolution to the main character's life problems after much bravery and cleverness. When they laughed and applauded at the end of the story I said 'Revenge seems to be something that is OK to think about' and they all agreed. It seemed that the fairy tale opened up the possibility, even acceptability, of discussion of these delicate topics with no feeling of shame or embarrassment. I could now bring in more 'serious readings' on those topics if the group wished, which they did.

I found that reading fairy tales answered the misplaced aggression problem in that it made difficult feelings accessible and not dangerous. It turned out to be a perfect way to keep the group balanced between 'serious' weeks and 'fairy tale' weeks, thus alleviating the attendance problem after a 'serious' session.

The advantage, in hindsight, to having men and women in the same group was that they began to develop compassion for each other, even when the other might be the same sex as the perpetrator of their abuse. They began to look beyond the surface appearance of things: not all people of the perpetrator's sex were by definition perpetrators. The issue of aggression came to the surface a lot more quickly and naturally in a mixed group. Once the women in the group saw that I did not crumble under attacks for bringing in the 'wrong' thing, they felt freer to admit to these once forbidden feelings. Men in the group learned that acting upon aggressive feelings might not always be the only option a person has. By examining how they were socialized to express themselves, they were able to learn from one another, sharing experiences with curiosity and compassion.

Making art the center of the group had many advantages. Art is often seen by the very literal-minded unconscious as a way of telling the story of what happened to the individual without breaking the 'never tell' rule set in place by the abuser. Art provides a tactile, physical outlet for stress which often surfaces quickly in this kind of group. The fact that it is tactile and physical and that they are in control of it is also a critical new experience for them. Individuals can interact verbally or not and they are still an active part of the group when they create artwork.

When the group members were in a creative mode, there was an openness to new possibilities, new ways of thinking that might not be there in a verbal group. It is openness to new things that this population needs, especially an openness to the idea that not everyone is an evil sorcerer capable of stealing others' power by simply touching them. They need an openness to the idea that if they choose to unlock Pandora's box, they can sort through things at their own pace. They can, in fact, lock and unlock the box as many times as they need to. They can take out one object, memory or feeling at a time, or they can keep taking out the same object, memory or feeling until they are ready to move on. The dissociative patient needs an openness to the idea that he is the creator of his life now. Some of the group members expressed surprise during the 'serious' weeks, hearing that what they thought were their personal symptoms, the things that labeled them mentally ill and set them apart from other people, were actually the only ways they had of coping with impossible situations. They began to empathize with themselves, or with the child they used to be.

This group was actually very successful. A second and third group were added before I left the center.

Dissociative patients and false memory

Baars and McGovern (1995) wrote an excellent article on false memory and traumagenic amnesia, entitled 'Steps toward healing: False memories and traumagenic amnesia may coexist in vulnerable populations'. They feel that child abuse is one of the most agonizing issues of our times. They criticize the tendency to polarize around the either/or dichotomy of 'recovered versus false memories', when both are likely to occur. They discuss some memory researchers' generalizations from mild stressors of the laboratory to the severe repeated traumas reported by abused populations. They believe that is an inferential leap that is not scientifically sound. They point out naturalistic studies that show some post-traumatic memory impairment, dissociativity (such as emotional numbing and detachment), but also increased suggestibility (the source of 'false memories'). They cite research that shows

20 percent of the normal population is highly suggestible and that in these individuals it is very easy to show suggested amnesia, detachment, perceptual blocking, etc., as well as to suggest dramatically false memories. They feel that adult survivors of abuse may show both more 'false memories' and more 'false forgetting' than the normal population.

When reading articles on 'false memories' I can't help but think of the individuals I have known who may be continuing to struggle to recover from early childhood trauma. I can't help but think of overcrowded inner-city mental health treatment facilities where therapists attempt to help them in the struggles. There are also administrators who may be worried about whether or not their agencies are going to be caught up in lawsuits over the implanting of false memories. Unfortunately, the climate within this culture is increasingly difficult for survivors of trauma.

Many mental health professionals have turned away from treating survivors out of fear of 'judicial accusations' (Acocella 1998, p.76). In 1993 Paul McHugh, director of psychiatry at Johns Hopkins University, called for an immediate end to multiple personality disorder treatment, suggesting that dissociation services be closed and patients dispersed to general psychiatric units.

The news and entertainment media, a vital aspect of this culture, has swung from supporting the survivor and the psychotherapist who works with them, to supporting those who have been accused of abuse and those suing therapists for implanting false memories. The media seems to swing in whatever way will bring in the most viewers or largest readership. If the public becomes bored and numb with survivors' tales, then the stories of wrongfully accused parents and destructive therapists are presented. I imagine the public will soon grow weary of these as well. Meanwhile, this embattled external climate seems to reflect the painful internal climate of the survivor. And if mental health workers and administrators are indeed following Paul McHugh's lead, the survivor is left without support. What, then, are we to do?

I think we need to consider the dissociative patient in a demystifying light. Symptoms such as disturbances in body image, a dissociated sense of self, a disrupted sense of history and causality, and a feeling of alienation from self and others can be seen as clearly related to the severe stresses these patients were put under as children. We need to consider the ameliorative effects of the creative process with dissociative patients, looking in depth at the specific and the detailed as well as the generalized and broader applications of using art making, puppet making and narrative. Perhaps we should explore using art to heal body image and sense of self, to create continuity of story (a sense of causality and history), and to build a community where individuals are able to feel joy and a hopefulness in being together.

Miscellaneous quotes

While working on this book, I reviewed some of the old videotapes of the puppetry group. In them I found these quotes:

> Most folks think we come up here and play with dolls. They have no idea. No idea at all.

> It's hard to know where the puppet ends and I begin. It's a very complicated thing.

> I just feel better when I'm up here. I think this is very subversive.

> When I think about life now, how good it is here in Puppetland, I realize it was dreams of how things would be that kept me alive in the Gulags. Now here we are, Vedrina and I, and little Nicholas, he is our dividend. We dreamed of this day. And Nicholas, he affirms our life. It is good. (Figure 8.1)

> Have a good life. You are good people. You deserve a good life.

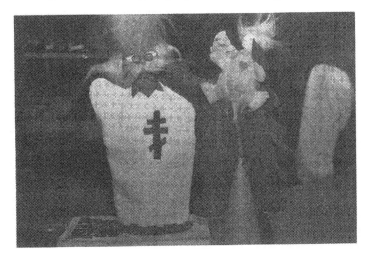

Figure 8.1 The family

And from Martin Buber:

> Rabbi Mendel said: 'I became a hasid because in the town where I lived there was an old man who told stories about zaddikim (leaders, those who stood the test). He told what he knew and I heard what I needed.' (Buber 1948, p.270)

> A rabbi, whose grandfather had been a disciple of the Baal Shem, was asked to tell a story. 'A story,' he said, 'must be told in such a way that it constitutes help in itself.' And he told; 'My grandfather was lame. Once they asked him to tell a story about his teacher. And he related how the holy Baal Shem used to hop and dance while he prayed. My grandfather rose as he spoke and he was so swept away by his story that he himself began to hop and dance to show how the master had done. From that hour on he was cured of his lameness. That's the way to tell a story!' (Buber 1947, pp.v–vi)

References

Abram, D. (1996) *The Spell of the Sensuous: Perception and Language in a More-Than-Human World.* New York: Pantheon Books.

Acocella, J. (1998) 'The politics of hysteria.' *The New Yorker LXXIV*, 7, 64–79.

Akhtar, S., Kramer, S. and Parens, H. (eds) (1996) *The Internal Mother: Conceptual and Technical Aspects of Object Constancy.* Northvale, NJ: Jason Aronson.

Aldridge, D. (1992) 'The needs of individual patients in clinical research.' *Advances 8*, 4, 58–65.

Aldridge, D. (1994) 'Single-case research designs for the creative art therapist.' *The Arts in Psychotherapy 21*, 5, 333–342.

Baars, B.J. and McGovern, K. (1995) 'Steps toward healing: False memories and traumagenic amnesia may coexist in vulnerable populations.' *Conscious Cognition 4*, 1, 68–74.

Balint, E. (1963) 'On being empty of oneself.' *International Journal of Psycho-Analysis 44*, 470–480.

Barker, P. (1985) *Using Metaphors in Psychotherapy.* New York, NY: Brunner Mazel Publishers.

Bass, E. and Davis, L. (1988) *The Courage to Heal: A Guide for Women Survivors of Child Sexual Abuse.* New York, NY: Harper Row.

Bergman, A. (1996) 'Mapping out the internal world.' In S. Akhtar, S. Kramer and H. Parens (eds) *The Internal Mother: Conceptual and Technical Aspects of Object Constancy.* Northvale, NJ: Jason Aronson.

Bettelheim, B. (1977) *The Uses of Enchantment: The Meaning and Importance of Fairy Tales.* New York, NY: Random House.

Bibring, E. (1953) 'The mechanism of depression.' In P. Greenacre (ed) *Affective Disorders.* New York, NY: International Universities Press.

Block, D. (1978) *So the Witch Won't Eat Me.* Boston: Houghton Mifflin.

Bly, R. (1988) *A Little Book on the Human Shadow.* San Fransisco: Harper Collins.

Bogdan, R.C. and Biklen, S.K. (1982) *Qualitative Research for Education; An Introduction to Theory and Methods.* Boston, MA: Allyn and Bacon.

Bower, T.A. (1977) *Primer of Infant Development.* San Francisco, CA: W.H. Freeman.

Bowlby, J. (1969) *Attachment and Loss, Volume 1.* New York, NY: Basic Books.

Bowlby, J. (1973) *Attachment and Loss, Volume 2.* New York, NY: Basic Books.

Bowlby, J. (1980) *Attachment and Loss, Volume 3.* New York, NY: Basic Books.

Bowlby, J. (1979) 'On knowing what you are not supposed to know and feeling what you are not supposed to feel.' *Canadian Journal of Psychiatry 24*, 403–404.

Braun, B.G. (ed) (1986) *The Treatment of Multiple Personality.* Washington, DC: American Psychiatric Press.

Briere, J.N. (1992) *Child Abuse Trauma: Theory and Treatment of the Lasting Effects.* Newbury Park, CA: Sage.

Brown, P.L. (1996) 'Life's thread stitched into quilts: An African-American art form is revived.' *The New York Times,* 4 April, Section C, p.1.

Bryant, D., Kessler, J. and Shirar, L. (1992) *The Family Inside: Working with the Multiple.* New York, NY: W.W. Norton.

Buber, M. (1947) *Tales of the Hasidim: The Early Masters.* New York, NY: Schoken Books.

Buber, M. (1948) *Tales of the Hasidim: The Later Masters.* New York, NY: Schoken Books.

Campbell, J. with Moyers, B. (1988) *The Power of Myth.* New York, NY: Doubleday.

Case, C. and Dailey, S. (eds) (1990) *Working with Children in Art Therapy.* London: Tavistock/Routledge.

Cash, T.F. and Pruzindky, T. (eds) (1990) *Body Images: Development, Deviance and Change.* New York, NY: The Guilford Press.

Cattanach, A. (1994) *Play Therapy: Where the Sky Meets the Underworld.* London: Jessica Kingsley Publishers.

Clegg, H. (1984) *The Reparative Motif in Child and Adult Therapy.* Northvale, NJ: Jason Aronson.

Clegg, H. (1995) *Reparation: Restoring the Damaged Self in Child and Adult Psychotherapy.* Northvale, NJ: Jason Aronson.

Cohen, B.M., Barnes, M. and Rankin, A.B. (1995) *Managing Traumatic Stress Through Art: Drawing from the Center.* Lutherville, MD: The Sidran Press.

Cohen, B.M. and Cox, C.T. (1995) *Telling Without Talking: Art as a Window into the World of Multiple Personality.* New York, NY: W.W. Norton.

Cohen, L., Berzoff, J. and Elin, M. (eds) (1995) *Dissociative Identity Disorder.* Northvale, NJ: Jason Aronson.

Combs, G. and Freedman, J. (1990) *Symbol, Story, and Ceremony; Using Metaphor in Individual and Family Therapy.* New York, NY: W.W. Norton.

Courtois, C.A. (1988) *Healing the Incest Wound: Adult Survivors in Therapy.* New York, NY: W.W. Norton.

Courtois, C.A. (1993) *Adult Survivors of Child Sexual Abuse.* Milwaukee, WI: Families International.

Demos, V (1985) 'Affect and the development of the self: A new frontier.' Self Psychology Conference, New York.

Deri, S. (1978) 'Transitional phenomena: Vicissitudes of symbolization and creativity.' In S. Grolnick and L. Barkin (eds) *Between Reality and Fantasy.* Northvale, NJ: Jason Aronson.

Deri, S. (1984) *Symbolization and Creativity.* New York, NY: International Universities Press.

Deutsch, R. (1959) *On the Mysterious Leap from the Mind to the Body.* New York, NY: International Universities Press.

Dissanayake, E. (1988) *What is Art For?* Seattle, WA: University of Washington Press.

Dolan, Y.M. (1991) *Resolving Sexual Abuse: Solution-Focused Therapy and Ericksonian Hypnosis For Adult Survivors.* New York, NY: W.W. Norton.

Du Rand, L. and Gerity, L. (1996) 'Puppetry: A collaboration between drama therapy and art therapy.' *Dramascope: The National Association for Drama Therapy Newsletter XVI,* 2, Summer/Fall, 9–10.

Edelstien, M.G. (1981) *Trauma, Trance and Transformation: A Clinical Guide to Hypnotherapy.* New York, NY: Brunner Mazel Publishers.

Eissler, K. (1962) *Leonardo da Vinci: Psychoanalytic Notes on the Enigma.* New York, NY: International Universities Press.

Engel, B. (1989) *The Right to Innocence: Healing the Trauma of Childhood Sexual Abuse.* Los Angeles, CA: Jeremy P. Tarcher.

Erickson, M. and Rossi, E. (1979) *Hypnotherapy: An Exploratory Casebook.* New York: Irvington.

Erskine, A. and Judd, D. (1994) *The Imaginative Body: Psychodynamic Therapy in Health Care.* Northvale, NJ: Jason Aronson.

Eth, S. and Pynoos, R.S. (eds) (1985) *Post-Traumatic Stress Disorder in Children.* Washington, DC: American Psychiatric Press.

Fenichel, O. (1945) *The Psychoanalytic Theory of Neuroses.* New York, NY: W.W. Norton.

Finkelhor, D. and Browne, A. (1986) 'Initial and long-term effects: A conceptual framework.' In D. Finkelhor (ed) *A Sourcebook on Child Sexual Abuse.* Beverly Hills, CA: Sage.

Finney, L.D. (1990) *Reach for the Rainbow: Advanced Healing for Survivors of Sexual Abuse.* New York, NY: The Putnam Publishing.

Fisher, S. and Cleveland, S. (1968) *Body Image and Personality.* New York, NY: Dover Press.

Fisher, S. (1986) *Development and Structure of the Body Image.* Hillsdale, NJ: Lawrence Erlbaum.

Fisher, S. (1990) 'The evolution of psychological concepts about the body.' In T. Cash and T. Pruzinsky (eds) *Body Images: Development, Deviance, and Change.* New York, NY: The Guilford Press.

Flannery, R.B. Jr. (1992) *Post-Traumatic Stress Disorder: The Victim's Guide to Healing and Recovery.* New York, NY: Crossroad.

Foster, P. (ed) (1994) *Minding the Body.* New York, NY: Doubleday.

Freud, S. (1905) 'Fragments of an analysis of a case of hysteria.' In J. Strachey (ed) *Standard Edition, Vol. 7.* London: The Hogarth Press, 1953.

Freud, S. (1920) 'Beyond the pleasure principle.' In J. Strachey (ed) *Standard Edition, Vol. 18.* London: The Hogarth Press, 1955.

Freud, S. (1923) 'The ego and the id.' *Standard Edition, Vol. 19.* London: The Hogarth Press, 1927.

Freud, S. (1924) 'The economic principle in masochism.' *Collected Papers, Vol. 2.* London: The Hogarth Press, 1933.

Freud, S. (1926) 'Inhibitions, symptoms, and anxiety.' In *International Psycho-analytical Library, 28.* London: The Hogarth Press, 1936.

Freytag, F.F. (1961) *Hypnosis and the Body Image.* New York, NY: The Julian Press.

Fuhrman, N.L. (1987) 'The developmental aspects of creative expression: implications in treatment of MPD [summary].' In B.G. Braun (ed) *Dissociative Disorders: Proceedings of the Third International Conference on Multiple Personality/Dissociative States.* Chicago, IL: Rush University.

Gardner, R.A. (1993) *Storytelling in Psychotherapy with Children.* Northvale, NJ: Jason Aronson.

Gediman, H. (1984) 'Actual neurosis and psychoneurosis.' *International Journal of Psycho-Analysis 65,* 195–202.

Gedo, M. (1985) 'The healing power of art: Goya as his own physician.' *Psychoanalytic Perspectives on Art 1,* 75–106.

Gendler, M. (1986) 'Group puppetry with school-age children: Rationale, procedure and therapeutic implications.' *The Arts in Psychotherapy 13*, 45–52.

Gerity, L.A. (1982) 'The Development of Body Image Through Art Therapy with an Autistic Child.' New York University, MA Thesis.

Gerity, L.A. (1997) *The Reparative Qualities of Art Therapy: Dissociative Identity Disorder and Body Image Development.* Ann Arbor, MI: UMI Dissertation Services.

Gil, E. (1991) *The Healing Power of Play: Working with Abused Children.* New York, NY: The Guilford Press.

Giovacchini, P.L. (1986) *Developmental Disorders: The Transitional Space in Mental Breakdown and Creative Integration.* Northvale, NJ: Jason Aronson.

Goldstein, J. and Kornfield, J. (1987) *Seeking the Heart of Wisdom: The Path of Insight Meditation.* Boston, MA: Shambhala.

Greenacre, P. (1958) 'Early physical determinants in the development of the sense of identity.' *Journal of American Psychoanalytic Association 6*, 612–627.

Greenacre, P. (1959) 'Play in relation to creative imagination.' *Psychoanalytic Study of the Child 14*, 61–80.

Greenacre, P. (1971) *Emotional Growth, Vol. 2.* New York, NY: International Universities Press.

Grolnick, S. and Barkin, L. (eds) (1978) *Between Reality and Fantasy: Transitional Objects and Phenomena.* New York, NY: Jason Aronson.

Grotstein, J. (1981) *Splitting and Projective Identification.* New York, NY: Jason Aronson.

Grotstein, J. (1986) 'The psychology of powerlessness: Disorders of self regulation and interactional regulation as a newer paradigm of psychopathology.' *Psychoanalytic Inquiry 6*, 93–118.

Harris, D. (1963) *Children's Drawings as Measures of Intellectual Maturity.* New York, NY: Harcourt, Brace and World.

Hartmann, H. (1964) *Essays in Ego Psychology.* New York, NY: International Universities Press.

Hedges, L.E. (1994) *Remembering, Repeating, and Working through Childhood Trauma: The Psychodynamics of Recovered Memories, Multiple Personality, Ritual Abuse, Incest, Molest, and Abduction.* Northvale, NJ: Jason Aronson.

Herman, J.L. (1992) *Trauma and Recovery: The Aftermath of Violence – From Domestic Abuse to Political Terror.* New York, NY: Basic Books.

Hoffer, W. (1949) 'Mouth, hand, and ego-integration.' *The Psychoanalytic Study of the Child 4*, 49–56.

Hoffer, W. (1950) 'Development of the body ego.' *The Psychoanalytic Study of the Child 5*, 18–23.

Irwin, E. and Rubin, J. (1976) 'Art and drama interviews: Decoding symbolic messages.' *The Arts in Psychotherapy, 3*, 169–175.

Jennings, S. and Minde, A. (1993) *Art Therapy and Drama therapy: Masks of the Soul.* London: Jessica Kingsley Publishers.

Johnson, S. (1987) *Humanizing the Narcissistic Style.* New York, NY: W.W. Norton.

Jones, E.E., Ghannam, J., Nigg, J.T. and Dyer, J. (1993) 'A paradigm for single-case research: The time series study of long-term psychotherapy for depression.' *Journal of Consulting and Clinical Psychology 61*, 3, 381–394.

Kabat-Zinn, J. (1990) *Full Catastrophe Living: Using the Wisdom of Your Body and Mind to Face Stress, Pain, and Illness.* New York, NY: Dell Publishing.

Kane, E. (1989) *Recovering from Incest: Imagination and the Healing Process.* Boston, MA: Sigo Press.

Kernberg, O. (1976) *Object Relations Theory and Clinical Psychoanalysis.* New York, NY: Jason Aronson.

Klein, M. (1921) 'The development of a child.' In *Love, Guilt and Reparation and Other Works, 1921–1945.* London: Hogarth, 1975.

Klein, M. (1929) 'Personification in the play of children.' In *Love, Guilt and Reparation and Other Works, 1921–1945.* London: Hogarth, 1975.

Klein, M. (1930) 'The importance of symbol-formation in the development of the ego.' In *Love, Guilt and Reparation and Other Works, 1921–1945.* London: Hogarth, 1975.

Klein, M. (1940) 'Mourning and its relation to manic-depressive states.' In *Contributions to Psycho-Analysis, 1921–1945.* London: The Hogarth Press, 1968.

Klein, M. (1945) 'The Oedipus complex in the light of early anxiety.' In *Contributions to Psycho-Analysis, 1921–1945.* London: The Hogarth Press, 1948.

Kluft, R. (ed) (1984) 'Six articles on MPD by Rome, Kluft, Wilbur, Braun, Caul, and Putnam.' *Psychiatric Annals 14,* 1.

Kluft, R. (1985a) 'The treatment of multiple personality disorder: Current concepts.' In F. Flach (ed) *Directions in Psychiatry, Vol. 5.* New York, NY: Hatherleigh.

Kluft, R. (ed) (1985b) *Childhood Antecedents of Multiple Personality.* Washington DC: American Psychiatric Press.

Kohut, H. (1977) *The Restoration of the Self.* New York, NY: International Universities Press.

Kluft, E. (ed) (1993) *Expressive and Functional Therapies in the Treatment of Multiple Personality Disorder.* Springfield, IL: Charles C. Thomas.

Kohut, H. (1985) *How Psychoanalysis Cures.* Hillside, NJ: The Analytic Press.

Koppelman, R. (1984) 'Hand puppetry with a chronic psychiatric population.' *The Arts in Psychotherapy 11,* 283–288.

Kornfield, J. and Feldman, C. (1996) *Soul Food: Stories to Nourish the Spirit and the Heart.* San Francisco, CA: HarperCollins.

Kramer, E. (1993) *Art as Therapy with Children, Second Edition.* Chicago, IL: Magnolia Street Publishers.

Kramer, E. (1996) 'Discussion of Kupfermann, K. The importance of lines.' *American Journal of Art Therapy 34,* 3, 62–74.

Kramer, S. and Akhtar, S. (eds) (1991) *The Trauma of Transgression: Psychotherapy of Incest Victims.* Northvale, NJ: Jason Aronson.

Kramer, S. and Salman, A. (eds) (1992) *When the Body Speaks: Psychological Meanings in Kinetic Clues.* Northvale, NJ: Jason Aronson.

Kris, E. (1952) *Psychoanalytic Explorations in Art.* New York, NY: International Universities Press.

Kris, E. (1955) 'Neutralization and sublimation.' *The Psychoanalytic Study of the Child 10,* 30–46.

Kris, E. (1975) *Selected Papers of Ernst Kris.* New Haven, CT: Yale University Press.

Kroll, J. (1993) *PTSD/Borderlines in Therapy: Finding the Balance.* New York, NY: W.W. Norton.

Krueger, D. (1984) *Success and the Fear of Success in Women*. New York, NY: The Free Press.

Krueger, D. (1988) 'Loss and restitution in eating disorder patients.' In D. Dietrich and P. Shabad (eds) *The Problem of Loss and Mourning: New Psychoanalytic Perspectives*. New York, NY: International Universities Press.

Krueger, D. (1989) *Body Self and Psychological Self: A Developmental and Clinical Integration of Disorders of the Self*. New York, NY: Brunner Mazel Publishers.

Krystal, H. (1978) 'Trauma and affects.' *Psychoanalytic Study of the Child 33*, 81–116.

Kuhns, R. (1983) *Psychoanalytic Theory of Art: A Philosophy of Art on Developmental Principles*. New York, NY: Columbia University Press.

Landy, R. (1986) *Drama Therapy: Concepts and Practices*. Springfield, IL: Charles C. Thomas.

Landy, R. (1983) 'The use of distancing in drama therapy.' *The Arts in Psychotherapy 10*, 175–185.

Lankton, C.H. and Lankton S.R. (1989) *Tales of Enchantment: Goal-Oriented Metaphors for Adults and Children in Therapy*. New York, NY: Brunner Mazel Publishers.

Levine, H.B. (ed) (1990) *Adult Analysis and Childhood Sexual Abuse*. Hillsdale, NJ: The Analytic Press.

Lichtenberg, J. (1978) 'The testing of reality from the standpoint of the body self.' *Journal of the American Psychoanalytic Association, 26*, 357–385.

Lichtenberg, J. (1985) *Psychoanalysis and Infant Research*. Hillsdale, NJ: The Analytic Press.

Linn, L. (1955) 'Some developmental aspects of the body image.' *International Journal of Psychoanalysis 36*, 36–42.

Lister, E. (1982) 'Forced silence: A neglected dimension of trauma.' *American Journal of Psychiatry 139*, 7, 872–876.

Mackay, B. (1987) 'A pilot study in drama therapy with adolescent girls who have been sexually abused.' *The Arts in Psychotherapy 14*, 1, 77–84.

Mahler, M. (1952) 'On child psychosis in schizophrenia: "Autistic and symbiotic infantile psychosis."' *Psychoanalytic Study of the Child 7*, 286–305.

Mahler, M. (1968) *On Human Symbiosis and the Vicissitudes of Individuation, Vol. 1*. New York: Jason Aronson.

Mahler, M., Pine, R. and Bergman, A. (1975) *The Psychological Birth of the Human Infant*. New York, NY: Basic Books.

Malchiodi, C.A. (1990) *Breaking the Silence: Art Therapy with Children from Violent Homes*. New York, NY: Bruner Mazel Publishers.

Marguiles, A. (1989) *The Empathic Imagination*. New York: W.W. Norton and Company.

McDevitt, J.B. (1996) 'The concept of object constancy and its clinical applications.' In S. Akhtar, S. Kramer and M. Parens (eds) *The Internal Mother: Conceptual and Technical Aspects of Object Constancy*. Northvale, NJ: Jason Aronson.

Meares, R. (1993) *The Metaphor of Play: Disruption and Restoration in the Borderline Experience*. Northvale, NJ: Jason Aronson.

Mills, J.C. and Crowley, R.J. (1986) *Therapeutic Metaphors for Children and the Child Within*. New York, NY: Brunner Mazel Publishers.

Murphy, P. (1994) 'The contributions of art therapy to the dissociative disorders.' *Art Therapy 11*, 1, 43–47.

Nichols, M.P. (1991) *No Place to Hide: Facing Shame so We Can Find Self-Respect*. New York, NY: Simon and Schuster.

Niederland, W. (1956) 'Clinical observations on the "little man" phenomenon.' *The Psychoanalytic Study of the Child 11*, 381–395.

Niederland, W. (1965) 'Narcissistic ego impairment in patients with early physical malformations.' *The Psychoanalytic Study of the Child 20*, 518–534.

Niederland, W. (1967) 'Clinical aspects of creativity.' *American Imago 24*, 6–33.

Ogden, T. (1986) *The Matrix of the Mind.* New York, NY: Jason Aronson.

Papousek, H. and Papousek, M. (1975) 'Cognitive aspects of preverbal social interaction between human infants and adults.' In Chicago Foundation Symposium *Parent–Infant Interaction.* New York, NY: Associated Scientific Publishers.

Peller, L. (1954) 'Libidinal phases, ego development, and play.' *Psychoanalytic Study of the Child 9*, 178–198.

Prior, S. (1996) *Object Relations in Severe Trauma: Psychotherapy of the Sexually Abused Child.* Northvale, NJ: Jason Aronson.

Putnam, F.W. (1989) *Diagnosis and Treatment of Multiple Personality Disorder.* New York, NY: The Guilford Press.

Rosal, M. (1987) 'Cognitive approaches in art therapy for children.' Presented at the 18th Annual National Conference of the American Art Therapy Association.

Rose, G. (1963) 'Body ego and the creative imagination.' *Journal of the American Psychoanalytic Association 11*, 775–789.

Rose, G. (1987) *Trauma and Mastery in Life and Art.* New Haven,CT: Yale University Press.

Rosenberg, E. (1949) 'Anxiety and the capacity to bear it.' *The International Journal of Psychoanalysis 30*, 1–12.

Ross, C.A. (1995) 'Current treatment of dissociative identity disorder.' In L. Cohen, J. Berzoff and M. Elin (eds) *Dissociative Identity Disorder.* Northvale, NJ: Jason Aronson.

Rossi, E.L. (1986) *The Psychobiology of Mind-Body Healing: New Concepts of Therapeutic Hypnosis.* New York, NY: W.W. Norton.

Roth, N. (1993) *Integrating the Shattered Self: Psychotherapy with Adult Incest Survivors.* Northvale, NJ: Jason Aronson.

Schacht, L. (1996) 'Winnicott's notion of the use of an object.' In S. Akhtar, S. Kramer and H. Parens (eds) *The Internal Mother: Conceptual and Technical Aspects of Object Constancy.* Northvale, NJ: Jason Aronson.

Schaefer, C.E. and Cangelosi, D.M. (1993) *Play Therapy Techniques.* Northvale, NJ: Jason Aronson.

Schilder, P. (1950) *The Image and Appearance of the Human Body.* New York, NY: International Universities Press.

Searles, H. (1979) 'Jealousy involving an internal object.' In J. LeBoite and A. Capponi (eds) *Advances in Psychotherapy of the Borderline Patient.* New York: Jason Aronson.

Segal, H. (1964) *Introduction to the Work of Melanie Klein.* New York, NY: Basic Books.

Segal, H. (1991) *Dream, Phantasy, and Art.* London: Routledge.

Segal, L. and Sendak, M. (1973) *The Juniper Tree and Other Tales from Grimm.* New York, NY: Farrar, Straus and Giroux.

Sgroi, S.M. (ed) (1988) *Vulnerable Populations, Vol. 2: Sexual Abuse Treatment for Children, Adults, Offenders, and Persons with Mental Retardation.* Lexington, MA: Lexington Books.

Sgroi, S.M. (ed) (1982) *Handbook of Clinical Interventions in Child Sexual Abuse.* Lexington, MA: Lexington Books.

Shapiro, M. (1988) *Second Childhood.* New York, NY: W.W. Norton.

Shengold, L. (1989) *Soul Murder: The Effects of Childhood Abuse and Deprivation.* New Haven, CT: Yale University Press.

Shirar, L. (1996) *Dissociative Children: Bridging the Inner and Outer Worlds.* New York, NY: W.W. Norton.

Silverman, L. (1979) 'The unconscious fantasy as therapeutic agent in psychoanalytic treatment.' *Journal of the American Academy of Psychoanalysis 7,* 189–218.

Silverman, L. and Weinberger, J. (1985) 'Mommy and I are one: Implications for psychotherapy.' *American Psychologist 40,* 1296–1308.

Smith, R.D., Buffington, P.W. and McCard, R.H. (1982) *Multiple Personality: Theory, Diagnosis, and Treatment: A Case Study.* New York, NY: Irvington Publishers.

Spitz, E. (1985) *Art and Psyche.* New Haven, CT: Yale University Press.

Spring, D. (1985) 'The visual language of multiplicity.' Presented at the 16th Annual National Conference of the American Art Therapy Association.

Spring, D. (1993) *Shattered Images: Phenomenological Language of Sexual Trauma.* Chicago: Magnolia Street Publishers.

Steinhardt, L. (1994) 'Creating the autonomous image through puppet theater and art therapy.' *The Arts in Psychotherapy 21,* 205–218.

Stern, D. (1985) *The Interpersonal World of the Infant.* New York, NY: Basic Books.

Stone, R. (1996) *The Healing Art of Storytelling; A Sacred Journey of Personal Discovery.* New York: Hyperion.

Thompson, R.F. (1983) *Flash of the Spirit.* New York, NY: Vintage Books.

Turner, V. (1974) *Dramas, Fields, and Metaphors: Symbolic Action in Human Society.* Ithaca: Cornell University Press.

Tyson, P. (1996) 'The development of object constancy and its deviations.' In S. Akhtar, S. Kramer and H. Parens (eds) *The Internal Mother: Conceptual and Technical Aspects of Object Constancy.* Northvale, NJ: Jason Aronson.

Van der Velde, C. (1985) 'Body images of one's self and of others: Developmental and clinical significance.' *Journal of the American Psychiatric Association 142,* 527–537.

Wallas, L. (1991) *Stories that Heal: Reparenting Adult Children of Dysfunctional Families using Hypnotic Stories in Psychotherapy.* New York, NY: W.W. Norton.

Waller, C. (1992) 'Art therapy with adult female incest survivors.' *Art Therapy 9,* 3, 135–138.

Webb, N.B. (1991) *Play Therapy with Children in Crisis.* New York, NY: The Guilford Press.

Wedding, D. and Corsini, R.J. (eds) (1989) *Case Studies in Psychotherapy.* Itasca, IL: F.E. Peacock Publishers.

White, M. and Epston, D. (1990) *Narrative Means to Therapeutic Ends.* New York, NY: W.W. Norton.

Wilson, J.P. (1989) *Trauma, Transformation, and Healing: An Integrative Approach to Theory, Research, and Post-Traumatic Therapy.* New York, NY: Brunner Mazel Publishers.

Wilson, L. (1987) 'Symbolism and art therapy: Theory and clinical practice.' In J.A. Rubin (ed) *Approaches to Art Therapy: Theory and Technique.* New York, NY: Brunner Mazel Publishers.

Wilson, L. (1993) 'Introduction to the second edition.' In E. Kramer, *Art as Therapy with Children.* Chicago, IL: Magnolia Street Publishers.

Winnicott, D. (1948) 'Reparation in respect of mother's organized defiance against depression.' In D.W. Winnicott *Collected Papers: Through Pediatrics to Psychoanalysis.* London: Tavistock, 1958.

Winnicott, D.W. (1949) 'Mind and its relation to the psyche-soma.' In D.W. Winnicott *Collected Papers: Through Pediatrics to Psychoanalysis.* London: Tavistock, 1958.

Winnicott, D.W. (1950–1955) 'Aggression in relation to emotional development.' In D.W. Winnicott *Collected Papers: Through Pediatrics to Psychoanalysis.* London: Tavistock, 1958.

Winnicott, D.W. (1965) *The Maturational Processes and the Facilitating Environment.* New York, NY: International Universities Press.

Winnicott, D.W. (1974) *Playing and Reality.* Harmondsworth: Penguin.

Winnicott, D.W. (1986) *Home is Where We Start From: Essays by a Psychoanalyst.* New York: W.W. Norton and Company.

Wisechild, L. (ed) (1991) *She Who Was Lost Is Remembered: Healing from Incest Through Creativity.* Seattle, WA: Seal Press.

Wolfenstein, M. (1966) 'Loss, rage, and repetition.' *The Psychoanalytic Study of the Child 24,* 432–460.

Workman, E. and Stillion, J. (1974) 'The relationship between creativity and ego development.' *The Journal of Psychology 88,* 191–195.

Yin, R.K. (1989) *Case Study Research: Design and Methods.* Newbury Park, CA: Sage.

Zipes, J. (trans.) (1987) *The Complete Fairy Tales of the Brothers Grimm.* New York, NY: Bantam Books.

Subject Index

abandonment 45, 50, 57, 79, 81
  depression 125
  of Jenny 26, 56
  Lani and Jenny interview on
    57–60
  transitional object for 42
abuse 13, 64–5, 67, 120, 124
  internalized 20
  puppet re-enactment of 102,
    106, 107
  sexual 10, 47, 56, 64
  in Steinberg case 105
  survivors 10, 64, 66, 126
Abuser (puppet) 100, 102, 103
abyss beneath Puppetland 97,
  103–4, 110
acceptance 60, 82, 118
advice for a mother 35–6
affect tolerance 41
agenda, psychiatrist's 37
agents of change 14, 16, 17, 18,
  21, 27
aggression 20, 72, 77, 129, 130
  Alexander's 90
  Jenny's 45, 50, 52, 54, 63, 80
aggressor, identification with 50,
  66, 79, 98
aggressor, Sally's role as 53
agoraphobia 90
alcoholism 90, 106
Alexander 89–96, 105–9, 115,
  118, 119
  as the Monster 113
alienation 120
amnesia 131, 132
annihilation 27
  anxiety 69, 71, 78, 79, 81
anorectics 130
anxiety 18, 20, 71, 75
  annihilation 69, 71, 78, 79,
    81
apprentice 118
arson 27, 60
  Lani and Carey interview on
    60–2
art room 8, 19, 24, 77, 80
  Jenny in the 23, 34, 79
art therapist 76, 77, 82, 120,
  126

in competition with music
  therapist 126
art therapy 13, 15, 69, 120,
  125–6
  Jenny's 27, 53, 78–86
  reparative qualities 17, 68, 84
art as a window 15, 36, 85
Artemis 96, 104, 119
arthritis 40, 41, 51, 63
aspirin 9, 26
attendance, issue of 127, 128,
  130

Baal Shem 134
baby bottle 29
baby monsters 113
baby, needy 36
baby puppet 105, 106, 107,
  108, 109
bad mother 78, 81, 108, 109,
  110
bad mother stuff 25
bad object 27, 71, 107, 120
barbed wire 23, 25
barriers 36
beachcomber 76
Beauty and the Beast 90
black tear 25
black and white 37, 44, 53, 72
body ego 73, 74, 78
body image 20–1, 73–8, 86,
  121, 129
  integrated 48, 120
  reparative qualities 16
  and weight 39
  whole 40, 82
body image representation 18,
  19, 73, 82, 86
  doll 40, 81, 121
  integration of 20, 120
  in Jenny's treatment 14, 85
body self 74–5
borderline individuals 71, 73,
  80, 89
Borderline–DID continuum 15
bottle, baby 29
boundaries 27, 74, 75, 78, 91
breast 23–4, 25, 80
Buddhist tale 87–8

caregiving 117
Carey 17, 26, 64, 73, 78
  aggression of 72
  described 29

destructiveness 40, 65
interviews with 36, 44, 47,
  48, 50, 51
  on arson and clay 60–3
Jenny's drawing of 84
and Joy 37
and the Monster 112–13
as object component 47
roles of 46
and Sweet Basil 53
Ceilidh house 117
change, agents of 14, 16, 17,
  18, 21, 27
child-abuse devil 106
childhood trauma 17, 64, 97,
  119, 120
City Dump 35, 80
clay 10, 23, 24, 55, 80, 82
  and Carey interview 60–2
cognitive distortion 64
cognitive functioning 64
comfort and security 23, 70, 78
community 86, 88, 110, 119
compartmentalization 66, 71
compassion 88, 103, 119
competition (between therapists)
  126
compulsion, unconscious 66–7
confusion 43, 50, 64, 66, 73
constructive tendencies 20
control 40, 64, 70, 72, 77, 127
cooperation 37
countertransference 16, 18, 97,
  125–7
creative arts therapists 20
creativity 63, 69, 76
  therapeutic value 75
crisis management 127
critic 40
Crystal 97, 98, 103–4
culture 76, 89, 124–5

day treatment center 19–20
  mental health 19–20
death wish 39, 52
defenses 70, 79, 119–20, 127
denial 70, 79
dependent relationships 38, 70
depressive position 72, 73
destructive urges 60, 77
devil, child-abuse 106
devil, transformed 107
dichotomous thinking 64–5, 66
differentiation 73, 75

disintegrated sense of self 21
dissociation 63–7, 79, 120, 129
  and false memory 131–2
  Jenny's identity 36, 79
Dissociative Identity Disorder or
  DID 13, 27, 36, 48, 72
doll/s 39–40, 42, 43, 48, 84
  see also puppets
  body image representation 40,
    81, 121
  making techniques 44–5
  young Jenny 51–6
dragon, dream 50, 53
drama therapist 105, 107, 108,
  120
drama therapy 67
drawing 18, 23, 44, 84, 85
  Lisa in 84
  projective 18, 74
dreams 50, 53, 54
drive theory 66

eating disorder 73
ego 46, 47, 73, 74, 78
emotional disturbance, types of
  9
empathy 66, 79, 91, 109, 131
Eric (psychiatrist) 29, 37, 50, 56,
  73
Eric (puppet) 29, 32, 52, 73,
  108, 109
  in drawing 84
ethnicity 73, 124–5
evil sorcerer, story of the
  129–30
external feedback 73

fairy tales 128, 129, 130
false memory 131–2, 132
  and dissociation 131–2
false self 65
fantasy 69, 70
fire setting see arson
fire-water 94
Fitcher's Feathered Bird 129,
  130
flexible boundaries 91
forbidden key 129
fossil memories 98, 109
fragmented identity 73

generativity 22, 75, 86
generic baby 105
generosity 14, 22, 111, 119
  of Rigvan 91, 96

and Wise Old Woman 117
giants, dream 53
good enough mother 18, 80, 89
good object 71, 85
  internalized 43, 116, 120,
    124, 125
good symbiotic mother 47, 48
grandmother 53
great-grandmother 50, 53–4,
    82, 116, 124
Greek Chorus 100, 101, 102,
    104, 106, 109
grief 82, 88
group/s 116, 118, 130
  mixed sex 130
  puppet-making 10, 19, 52,
    68, 80, 83
    description of 27, 29
  survivor's art group 68,
    127–31

headache 46, 58
healing metaphors 86
helplessness 40, 41, 43
historical subject 72
holding environment 77, 79, 81,
  82, 83
  maternal 69, 72, 76, 78
homework 43
hope 43, 51, 53, 82, 87
Hound Dog 34, 35

identification with the aggressor
  50, 66, 79, 98
identity 47, 65, 67, 73
  projective identification 21,
    70, 79, 80, 120
imagination 21, 67, 77, 89
imaginative play 27, 76
independence 38, 47, 56, 123,
  125
Indra's net 67
infant needs 69
inner child 128
inner dialogue 38
inner representations 67, 73, 74,
  84
inner space 77
integrated body schema 74
integrated identity 73
integration 14, 20, 21, 48, 71,
  120
  of psyche and soma 76
  of self in community 86

internal object world 83, 84, 98
internalization 20, 21, 49,
  120–1, 125
  development of 74
  and Jenny 54, 57, 80, 105
internalized bad mothers 108,
  109
internalized bad object 107, 120
internalized good object 43,
    116, 120, 124, 125
internalized object world 68, 84
internalized objects 69, 109,
    110, 120
internalized traumata and abuse
  20
interviews 35–6, 125
introjected mother 75
introjection 70, 79
intrusive thoughts 64
intuit 38, 48
Iron John 113

Jenny
  background 9–10, 13–14, 17
  case of 23–62, 105–10, 119,
    123–4
    art therapy 27, 53, 78–86
    behavior in pottery room
      23, 36, 53, 79
    and the Monster 113
  chart 26–7, 38
  journal see journal
  Little Jenny 54, 55, 124
  as puppeteer 14, 36, 84, 85
  separate personality 64, 73
journal 38, 41, 43, 45, 52–4, 56
  comments on 65, 84
  described 37
Joy 17, 46, 65, 72, 73, 126
  creation of 29
  drawing of 84
  interviews with (taped) 36, 37,
    45
  Little Joy 53, 54, 55, 56, 124
judicial accusations 132
Jungian personal unconscious
    109, 110
kids 54, 56
kiln 20, 81, 123
knight in shining armor 48

Ladder to the Moon 88
Lani 45, 49, 56, 57–62
life events 87

Lisa (puppet) 29, 32, 49, 73
Lisa, Dr 29, 49, 50, 54, 73
Lita 32, 35, 73, 84
Little Carey 54, 55, 56, 84, 124
Little Jenny 54, 55, 124
Little Joy 53, 54, 55, 56, 84,
   124
log-keeping 36–7
long bag, Bly's 109–10
loss 60, 110, 115–19, 125
   acceptance of 60, 82, 118

malignant negative identity 65
Margaret (puppet) 32, 84, 104,
   105–10, 123
Margaret, Jenny's mother 46, 51,
   63, 78–9, 124
masochism 41, 46
masochistic stance 38, 39, 47
maternal holding environment
   69, 72, 76, 78
Measle 98, 101, 102, 103
media 132
memory 38, 117, 131, 132
mental compartmentalization 66
mental health day treatment
   center 19–20
mental illness 9, 14, 15, 131
merging 39, 78, 104
metaphor 14, 72, 87, 95, 126
   art 36, 52, 126
   Bly's bag 109
   healing 86
   visual 34
metaphoric language 100, 103
metaphoric level of therapy 105,
   106
migraine 26, 37, 40, 41, 63
mirroring 74, 76, 81
Miss Pie 101, 102
missymbolization 71
mixed sex groups 130
Monster (puppet) 104, 110, 111
   tale of the 112–13, 114
monsters, baby 113
monsters, dream 53
mother, bad 78, 81, 108, 109,
   110
mother, borderline 89
mother, good enough 18, 80, 89
mother, introjected 75
mother salamander 82
mother, symbiotic 47, 48
mourning 72, 115, 125

Mr Mad 34, 35, 41–2, 50, 80,
   84
   described 32, 81
multidimensional web identity
   47
multiple identity 47
multiple personality disorder see
   Dissociative Identity
   Disorder
mural 110, 111, 117
murderous fantasy 67
music 57, 60, 64, 68, 82, 126
music therapist 57, 60, 64, 68,
   82
   in competition with art
      therapist 126
   directive 85, 126
music therapy 37, 123, 126
mythic plane 87, 89, 115

narcissism 73, 74, 80
narrative 86, 119
narrative therapy 87, 88
needs 32, 50, 69
negative projection 18
nervousness 56
'never tell' 131
Nicholas 133
numbing and detachment 131

object constancy 72, 73, 88, 96,
   125, 126
object relations 21, 46, 67–73,
   81, 125
object-component 46, 47
objets trouvés 76
oral sex 57
osteoporosis 41, 51, 63

paintings 85
Pandora's box 128, 131
panic attack 50
papier-mâché 39, 42, 75, 81
paranoid schizophrenia 27, 69,
   72
parent, bad/good 66
parental abuse 64
parental attention 66
parental role 98
part objects 71, 72, 73
parts of self 71, 72
patchwork blankets 52
patchwork quilt 51, 54, 55, 56,
   57, 82, 125
patients 13, 15, 19, 86

borderline 71, 73, 80
pencil holder 24, 80
perpetrator 39, 98, 130
persecutory objects 72, 73, 75
personality disorder 13
phallic finger puppet 32
phantasy 69, 70
pinch pots 40
playing alone in the presence of
   the mother 76
playspace 76, 77
pleasure 23, 45, 75
population, patient 13, 15, 19
positive feelings 16, 51, 52, 56
post traumatic stress disorder 13
potential space 76, 82
pottery room 20, 80, 81
   Jenny's behavior in 23, 36,
      53, 79
power 16, 57, 66, 103, 129,
   131
preconscious level 129
preverbal imagery 17
preverbal reparation 17
prohibition 38
projection 18, 70, 79, 104, 110
projective drawing 18, 74
projective identification 21, 70,
   79, 80, 120
psychiatrist puppet 38, 73
psychiatrist's agenda 37
psychic synthesis 67
psychoanalytic theory 73
psychological integration 14
psychological self 74–5
psychosomatic disease 40–1, 49
psychotherapy 11
puppet-making 14, 27, 93
   group 10, 19, 52, 68, 80, 83
   described 27, 29
   therapeutic value 84, 86
puppeteer/s 85, 86, 100, 102,
   119, 124
   reunions 124
Puppetland 89, 91, 98, 103,
   114
   anything could happen in 89
   puppets 84–5
   see also doll/s
   ethnic race 73, 124
pyromania 130

quilt, patchwork 51, 54, 55, 56,
   57, 82, 125

rage, self-protective 89
Ralph 45, 46
rape 26, 39, 45, 47
rationalizing abuse 64
reading 55, 127, 128
reconciliation 108, 109
redemption 98, 105, 109
reintegration 117
reinternalization 70
remorselessness 109
reparation 14, 60, 67, 69, 82
    defined 20–1
    reparation and loss 115–19
    theory 77–8
reparative narrative 86
reparative qualities
    art therapy 15, 17, 68, 75, 84
    body image 16
representation 27, 41, 53, 73–5, 82
    body image 19, 77
    self representation 14, 73, 125
representational world 65–6, 69, 78, 79
rescue 66
restorative actions 77
retraumatize 127, 128
retribution 41
Rigvan 106, 107, 108, 115, 116, 118
    generosity of 91, 96
    story of 91–5
role/s 40, 46, 53, 64, 69, 98
    Jenny as puppeteer 14, 36, 84, 85
Rutherford (dream dragon) 53

sabotage 41
sadistic concepts 20, 46, 47, 64
Sally 37, 38, 123
    relationship with Jenny 39, 47, 48, 50, 56, 63
    Sally's dog 41, 52, 53
sanctuary 68, 90
satisfaction 23, 37, 38, 75
Sebastian 32, 84
security and comfort 23, 70, 78
seduction 66
self constancy 73
self representation 14, 73, 125
self-component 46, 47
self-esteem 46
sense of self 85, 120
    healthy 14, 74, 86

separate personality, Jenny's 64, 73
separation 39, 60, 87
sexual abuse 10, 47, 56, 64
shades of gray 44, 50, 53, 72
shadow, collective 105, 109, 110, 113, 114
shape-shifters 103
Siberian work camps 91
silence 38, 39
slab work 40, 49, 83
somatization 39, 40, 46, 49
something 55
soothe 18, 49, 53
soothing 40, 60, 70, 80
sorrow 73, 89, 92, 107, 115
split world 71, 98, 128
splitting 40, 70, 71, 72, 79
    and transference 126
Steinberg, Lisa, case of 105
Stewart (therapist) 68
sublimation 38, 68, 69, 95, 120, 121
subversive qualities 95, 133
suggestibility 132
suicide 26, 37, 38, 107
super-ego 46, 75
survivor 64, 66, 70, 126, 132
    adult 13, 22, 64, 68, 70, 85
    childhood sexual abuse 10, 64
    holocaust 107
survivor's art group 68, 127–31
Susan 97, 98–103, 109, 110
Sweet Basil 42, 43, 51, 52, 53, 56
    concern for Jenny 45, 49
    quilt for 57
    as transitional object 84, 124, 125
symbiotic contentment 24
symbiotic state 48, 79
symbolism 21, 69, 71, 74, 75, 80
systems theory 67

talisman 116, 119
tape recorded interviews 35, 36
therapists
    creative arts 20
    directive 85, 126
    drama 105, 107, 108, 120
    music 57, 60, 64, 68, 82, 126
Toddler 98, 100, 101, 102
Tomboy 98, 101, 102, 103

toxins 80
transference 18, 97, 102, 104, 126
    diluted 102, 104
transformation 80, 81, 87, 107
transitional objects 16, 77, 120, 124, 125
    first 74
    Jenny's own 82, 84
transitional space 16, 76, 77, 78, 89, 118
trauma 13, 20, 46, 65, 66
    childhood 17, 64, 97, 119, 120
traumagenic amnesia 131
traumatic experience 76
treatment, examination of 78–86
tribe 86, 92, 115, 117

Ukraine 91
ulcer 40
unconscious compulsion 66–7
unconscious, figurative 84
unconscious functioning 47
unconscious level 129
unconscious, literal-minded 130
unconscious processes 75
unconscious, work on 128
Ungar 92, 93, 106, 115, 116, 119

Vedrina 91–3, 94–5, 116, 133
verbal therapy 13, 17, 18
vestigial memory 117
Victoria 92, 116

weight, body 39, 41, 51, 54, 55–6, 63, 126
wheelchair 41, 51, 123
whole body image 40, 82
whole-object 72, 73
whole-object relationships 73, 81, 125
Winter, Paul 111
winter solstice celebration 104, 110, 117
Wise Old Woman 112, 116, 117, 118, 119, 125
    hearth mural 110
writing 38, 43

Xena (planet) 103

zaddikim 134

Author Index

Abram, D. 78
Acocella, J. 132
Akhtar, S. 73
Angyal, A. 52

Baars, B.J. 131
Balint, E. 78
Bass, E. 127
Bergman, A. 72
Bettelheim, B. 95, 128
Bloch, D. 78
Bly, R. 109, 113
Bower, T.A. 21
Briere, J.N. 64, 65, 66
Buber, M. 134

Clegg, H. 20, 77, 78

Davis, L. 127
Deri, S. 71, 76, 77
Du Rand, L. 93, 115, 116, 125

Epston, D. 87, 88
Erickson, M. 128

Federn, E. 9
Fenichel, O. 74
Finney, L.D. 127
Freud, S. 20, 21, 40, 41, 73

Gerity, L. 10, 11, 27, 34, 37,
    45, 46, 47, 49, 50, 51,
    52, 53, 56, 60, 62, 81,
    93, 124
Giovacchini, P.L. 21, 77
Goldstein, J. 88
Grotstein, J. 21

Herman, J.L. 17, 64, 65, 90

Klein, M. 11, 20, 21, 23, 72, 77
Kluft, R. 27
Kornfield, J. 88
Kramer, E. 18, 21, 68, 120
Kramer, S. 73
Krueger, D. 18, 73, 74, 75, 85
Krystal, H. 40, 41, 49

Landy, R. 67
Lankton, C.H. and Lankton, S.R.
    87, 91, 95
Lister, E. 38, 39, 48

Mahler, M. 11, 72, 75
Margulies, A. 75, 77
McGovern, K. 131
McHugh, P. 132

Niederland, W. 20

Ogden, T.H. 21, 46, 47, 69, 70

Parens, H. 73
Prior, S. 67

Rosal, M. 43
Rossi, E. 128

Searles, H. 47
Segal, H. 23
Segal, L. 129
Sendak, M. 129
Shapiro, M. 52
Shengold, L. 11, 64, 65, 66, 67,
    72, 75, 86
Stone, R. 88

Turner, V. 87, 88

White, M. 87, 88
Wilson, D. Laurie 21, 41
Winnicott, D.W. 11, 21, 76, 89

Milton Keynes UK
Ingram Content Group UK Ltd.
UKHW032021121024
449584UK00006B/96